How to Avoid Dialysis and Cure Kidney Disease

BY
TERRY COOKSEY

COVER ART
BY
TERRY COOKSEY

ISBN-13: 978-1-939147-11-0

ISBN-10: 1-939147-11-5

How to Avoid Dialysis and Cure Kidney Disease

Table of Contents

ISBN-13: 978-1-939147-11-0

ISBN-10: 1-939147-11-5

All Rights Reserved – 2012 © American Publishing US

1 -Introduction

Congratulations on finding this book! You are about to embark on saving your own life and significantly improving your health and avoiding dialysis; on your way to most likely curing yourself. In this book you will find the information you need to do all of this. I tell how you can avoid dialysis by contacting the only Doctor in the country that has helped over a thousand people to avoid dialysis through his drug treatments, which have been clinically proven to work.

And for those who wish to take responsibility for their own health, and for those whose Creatinine is above 3.9, I give you the complete story and details about how I became the first person in America to reverse my chronic kidney disease and cure myself. And what I did, not only cured my chronic kidney disease, but cured me of every disease and medical condition I had. I cured myself of 20+ years of arthritis, intestinal bleeding, bleeding gums, headaches and heartburn.

I also cured myself of an enlarged heart and gout; as well as pulling myself back from the brink of diabetes. But my first experience with curing chronic "incurable" disease was in 1996, when I cured myself of "incurable" bladder stones after four excruciatingly painful attacks in just 3 or 4 years. I did so without doctors, by taking magnesium oxide and Vitamin C.

As a matter of fact, I cured myself after stopping my fourth bladder stone attack WHILE it was in progress! I took 2 400mg magnesium oxide tablets about an hour after the fourth attack started. And within 45 minutes, the attack began to fade away, and that was the end of it. No one was more shocked than I was. I have kept taking magnesium since then to insure I would not have any more bladder stones, or develop kidney stones or bone spurs. And I did it with proven science, which doctors refuse to be interested in.

So I am shoutin' from the roof tops about what I did, so that the cure for chronic kidney disease and all disease can be brought to an end, or at least a bare minimum. I celebrate still being alive every day by talking about what cured me. And what cured me is written in this book for you to follow and cure yourself. I can only tell you that you WILL cure yourself, because that is the only way I know. But since I do not know all the different situations people face in having kidney disease, some

MAY not be cured. But the least you will achieve is significantly improving your health and adding days, weeks and years to your life. And that's something you can't get from doctors.

In this book I will tell you how to contact Dr. Moskowitz to participate in his drug treatments which will enable you to avoid dialysis and put your chronic kidney disease in check. But even though Dr. Moskowitz's drug treatments have been proven in clinical trials and that data given to the National Institute of Health, they have refused to do their basic duty of sending that information out to the medical profession. You would think they would be interested in saving lives and saving some of that $50 billion a year that the government spends on dialysis and Medicare and Medicaid payments for patients with chronic kidney disease. But they aren't interested in the least bit. And have refused to get the data from Dr. Moskowitz to the medical community. And these cold hearted monsters are not alone in this gruesome behavior!

When I was searching the INTERNET to begin writing this book, I did a Google search for avoiding dialysis to see if anyone had finally written a book about avoiding dialysis or curing chronic kidney disease. And whose web site came up almost at the top? A site/company called Davita. I clicked the link and it took me to a forum discussion board for kidney patients.

I couldn't find anything about avoiding dialysis on their site forum. So I started a topic about me curing myself of chronic kidney disease. But as posters began to attack and ridicule me for this, I began to question whether that site had anything to do with helping kidney patients. As I backed up on the URL and go to the root/home page of that forum, it turned out to be a company that provides dialysis services for kidney patients. And it was no surprise when this heartless, immoral dialysis company banned me from their site permanently just 3 days later!

The vicious intolerance of cures by the entire medical profession is an ugly, but real thing. But let's not pick on heartless Davita.com. Heck, I sent emails with detailed information to the National Kidney Foundation about me reversing and curing myself of chronic kidney disease. And I haven't heard one little peep from them; not even a congratulations on being cured from them! All these hypocrites are just support for the failed medical profession. But are of no value to anyone who wishes to get better or be cured! But my first experience with this vicious heartless attitude of doctors and the medical profession came from my own doctors. And it only took them about 18 months to show me they are intolerable of anyone getting better or curing themselves.

The doctors that diagnosed me with chronic kidney disease ended up throwing me out of their clinic, refusing to be my doctors any more. Once they saw me improve on my own without any help from them for my kidneys, they sent me certified letters stating they would no longer be my doctors. I kept those letters in case they claim this is not true. I started off with those doctors and clinic with my Creatinine at 2.9 and climbing to 3.1 two months later; on course for the 0.1 monthly rise in Creatinine that leads all kidney patients to the dialysis machine. Those doctors got their first proof that I was doing what they had never done, when my lab results came back 5 months later and my Creatinine was down to 2.6. Then when my lab tests came back 11 months after that and my Creatinine was down to 2.2, they knew I was curing myself or at least reversing my kidney disease with a sustained remission. Barely six weeks later, I get those certified letters stating that my 2 doctors would no longer be my doctors.

It was during the next months following me receiving those certified letters, that I found Dr. Moskowitz's GenoMed site and contacted him. So because of that, I was so glad those worthless doctors of Death and dialysis did me a favor by kicking me out of their clinic and refusing to be my doctors. I will be talking about Dr. Moskowitz in Chapter 3 about Dr. Moskowitz's drug treatments, and also toward the end of Chapter 8. If you have the printed version of this book or a PDF version, then you can check the Index for Dr. Moskowitz. But why did I tell you this about doctors and the medical profession?

I did it for a few reasons. First, it's no secret that there is no cure for chronic kidney disease in the medical profession. So if you want to be cured, then doctors and the medical profession are NOT of any value with that, because doctors never studied cures in Medical school. So they can't cure you and don't even have any interest in curing you. You need the medical profession to do what they actually do – take tests and diagnostics and prescribe drugs. If you are going to cure yourself or improve your health that is something you are going to have to do on your own. And to do that, you must empower yourself with the knowledge that will cure you or at least greatly improve your health.

That fact excites me every time I think about it! You have no hope. There is no cure. Doctors can't do a thing to help your kidneys get better. In just a very short time, you will be on the dialysis machine as you wait for a possible kidney transplant that may or may not work. And as the symptoms slowly increase and progress, you must decide when dialysis could be better than continuing to suffer with all the symptoms you have. And until Dr. Moskowitz started helping people avoid dialysis for years, the only help kidney patients had was Dr. Mackenzie Walser's book Coping With Kidney Disease – A 12 Step Program to Help You Avoid Dialysis; which was to learn Dr. Walser's low 20 gram daily protein diet to arrest the progression of chronic kidney disease.

That is all the help I ever found in all the hours I spent trying to find anything that might or would help my kidneys. And I know just about all of you with chronic kidney disease are going through these same difficulties and hopelessness from doctors and the medical profession. You don't have the time to waste with being mad at or trusting doctors, you are going to die very soon unless YOU do something about it.

Most people have told me that "God gave you the sense to know to go to the doctor." But I tell them that's the problem. Your "God" didn't give you the sense to know to go to the doctor and get a cure, OR LOOK ELSEWHERE until you found a cure!!!!!" And that is the beginning of the attitude changes you have to make in order to cure yourself. And since poisons in our food, drinks and water supplies cause all disease, you can learn to avoid those poisons that caused your disease, and cure yourself on your own. And you can do it WHILE you still go to your doctors who have no cures. Another attitude you must change is about cures.

Your present attitude about cures is that there is no cure. There are no cures. But how about facing the fact that there is a cure for every disease known to man, but they're all OUTISIDE the medical profession. But the great thing is that you can afford the cures. What you cannot afford is the treatments for your disease, as you are led down the path to dialysis and Death. And dialysis costs $100,000 a year per patient.

So start changing your way of thinking and remember that there is a cure for every disease. You just have to take the time to find it. This book focuses on the millions of people with the same disease I cured myself of. But no matter what disease you have, doing what Chapters 5, 6 and 7 tell you to do, will improve your health and most likely cure you of any disease you have. And that means all the diseases doctors pretend are "incurable". Make cures a part of your daily thinking and work to make cures a part of your life and the lives of your family and other loved ones.

So you **train yourself to remember there is a cure for every disease known to man. And you look for those cures until you find them. And you keep cures a part of your life from now on! You know what a CURE is? A CURE is the thing that saves your life from sickness and disease.**

But when it comes to the United States, the key to curing yourself of any and all disease is by reducing and eventually eliminating as much of the poisons you consume through food, drinks and unfiltered water, as you possibly can. And that's what this book is mainly about. But you'll need at least one more attitude adjustment to see these facts clearly. That's because you actually trust the FDA.

Yes, it's the FDA that says all these disease causing, addicting poisons are "safe". The FDA is also the ones who claim those prescription drugs that kill at least 25,000 Americans each year are "safe". The FDA claims all these poisons are "safe" as long as they don't kill you right away. You already know your parents told you poisons are harmful! But you forgot that because the FDA says poisons are safe as long as they're in your food, drinks and water. The solution is simple. Stop believing that poisons are safe and start learning what these poisons are, find them in your food and drinks, wherever they are. And avoid them. But be warned – once you start doing this, the grocery store gets smaller and smaller.

I can only think about all of you who are about to get started doing what this book says to do, and save your lives and add so much more time to your lives, and be excited for you. Oh how I WISH I had this book to help me when I was dying, on the road to dialysis in just months. So I am so thrilled to provide for all of you, the information I needed to save my life, avoid dialysis and become the first person in this country to cure myself of chronic kidney disease. And lucky for you, I did not include hardly anything that did NOT work (except for doctors and the medical profession).

I will tell you up front that much of this book is taken from an earlier book of mine titled Self-Care HealthCare Guide. If you have any disease besides kidney disease, you will want to get that book for information on specific things you can do to greatly improve your health and cure yourself of each specific disease. I could just about take Chapters 5, 6 & 7 and build a book for each and every disease around those chapters.

This is due to the huge fact that poisons cause all disease except the 20% caused by germs and viruses.

Please feel free to write us and tell us your story about how you cured yourself or greatly improved your health or about you avoiding dialysis because of what you read and learned in this book.

If you want to reduce the number of pages you read and still get all the help you need, just skip Chapter 8. That Chapter is just about my experiences I had with the medical profession after developing CKD. Such a tiny trickle of help came from all that time and money spent with them.

2 - You're Probably Dying, So Let's Get You Some Help

Let me say this very clearly and as strongly as I can. This book has NO GIMMICKS. This book presents scientific facts that give the results stated in this book. It is up to YOU to take these scientific facts about your body, disease and the food, drinks and water you consume, and put that science to work for you, to train and force your body to heal itself naturally. Basically, you learn to recognize the saturation of poisons in your food, drinks and water, in order to avoid, reduce and eliminate those poisons. You should drink plenty of pure clean water. Correct your major nutrient deficiencies. And fast as often as possible to speed your healing along. A fast of 12-16 hours is easy to achieve on a regular basis

If you got this book, then you are probably dying right now. So you need to get right to the facts that are going to keep you off dialysis and cure your chronic kidney disease. I know I searched many many hours and days for any little shred of information that might help my kidneys get better. But there is little information in the world that can help you. The main reason is because no one has had any success in helping kidney patients get better or cured. You went to the doctor and he told you that you have kidney disease and that there is no cure for it. They tell you that you will progressively get worse and eventually die from your kidney disease. And that all they can do is help you with the symptoms of chronic kidney disease as they develop.

The typical story for a kidney patient is that they first have elevated levels of Creatinine and BUN in their blood. But the first sign of trouble is usually a problem with Potassium (K). Your muscles will become tight and give you cramps if you're low on Potassium. And if your Potassium is too high, you will experience heart palpitations which are life threatening. Your heart pounds out of control. If your blood pressure is high, you will bruise easily. As your Creatinine rises at the rate of 0.1 each month, you began to get swelling in your ankles and face from the water not being properly controlled. Your skin begins to itch more and more. And by the time your Creatinine reaches 5.0+ 2-3 years after getting chronic kidney disease, you have to decide WHEN you want to start dialysis.

One thing you have to decide is who you are going to listen to? Are you going to continue listening to the doctors who have no cures and won't do anything to help your kidneys get better? OR, you going to listen to someone like me who did what no doctors have ever done, and cured myself of chronic kidney disease? I wrote a book about this called Self-Care Health Care Guide. But I didn't restrict the information in that book to just curing chronic kidney disease. But the cure for chronic kidney disease is also the basic cure for almost all disease. So I am writing this book to concentrate on the 30 Million Americans that have chronic kidney disease and anyone and everyone else in the world that has this always fatal disease.

You don't realize the value of your kidneys until you get kidney disease. Then you don't understand what is happening to you. I want to talk about that right now, but later I will go into exactly what happened to me as I hopelessly tried to get the medical profession to help my kidneys get better. The doctors even made remarks on my medical records implying that I am crazy because I kept asking them what they were going to do to help my kidneys and I kept telling them I was going to be cured. So the medical profession is a two-edged sword.

You naturally turn to the medical profession to find out what is wrong with you after you get sick and habitually feel bad. **The medical profession is very helpful in diagnosing diseases. They are the exclusive source for prescription drugs, lab tests, surgeries, treatments for sickness and medical procedures. But the things that they can't help you with are cures and medicine. They don't teach cures in their medical schools, so doctors never learn the cures that have been around for centuries. And all the medicines man had were herbs. Herbs are merely plants that have been used as medicines. That classifies and defines them as herbs.**

But yet no doctors in the modern medical profession has studied medicine; herbs. My doctor told me outright that he didn't know a thing about herbs (medicine). And it doesn't matter to any doctors that they swore an oath to Hippocrates, the Father of Medicine, whose practice was founded on herbs and fasting. But I am not telling you to do without doctors. I am clarifying what doctors CAN and CAN NOT do for you.

You will need some of their drugs for high blood pressure and maybe a thing or two besides. And you will need them to test your blood to see how well your cure is coming along and that your Creatinine level is no longer increasing. You may want to get an Ultrasound if you are paying cash and a CT Scan if your insurance will pay for it.

But the first thing your doctor will do if you seem to have kidney problems is determine whether or not your kidney problems are being caused by kidney stones. **So before I give you the information on How to**

Avoid Dialysis and Cure (chronic) Kidney Disease, let's see if your kidney problems are caused by kidney stones. Then I'll give you the cure for kidney stones.

What If My Kidney problem is Kidney stones?

The first thing doctors will look into if there is a problem with your kidneys found in your blood tests, is to see if you have kidney stones. If you have kidney stones, you can either dissolve them naturally or have them surgically removed.

Kidney stones are cured the same way bladder stones and bone spurs are cured. The one factor that makes kidney stones different is the effect of uric acid in forming uric acid kidney stones. Over production of Uric acid is what causes gout. But its role in forming kidney stones is what separates the cure for uric acid kidney stones from calcium based kidney stones, bladder stones and bone spurs.

Too much Uric acid for prolonged periods of time leads to uric acid stones. Uric acid is produced when purines break up. Purines are found in foods like meat, peas, beans, liver and some alcoholic drinks. So avoid a diet high in animal protein. It is very important to drink a lot of water to help prevent and cure kidney stones. You can't allow excess uric crystals to remain in the kidneys and form these uric acid stones. Drinking 2-3 quarts of pure water a day will help pass around 90% of kidney stones. So don't forget! Adding pH drops to the water and drinking baking soda and water is even better.

And don't forget the magnesium, if you have calcium kidney stones, which will dissolve this most common type of kidney stones. B6 also acts like magnesium in the body. The science this cure comes from is that magnesium is needed in the body to dissolve calcium so that calcium can be used by your body. If you don't have enough magnesium, these undissolved calcium particles are free to bind to toxins(free radicals, poisons) to form stones in your kidneys; as well as in your bladder. You need antioxidants such as Vitamins C, A & E; as well as lesser known antioxidants like Selenium and Alpha Lipoic Acid and others to remove toxins from your body, and the magnesium to dissolve calcium. This one-two punch of vitamin supplementation can cure you of calcium based kidney and bladder stones and bone spurs.

To cure yourself of these calcium based kidney stones, you need to take at least 800mg magnesium oxide and 3000-5000mg Vitamin C daily until cured. The stones will dissolve slowly over a short period of time because of the excess magnesium; perhaps 6-8 weeks, or longer if the stones are bigger than usual. And by taking the magnesium oxide, over 300 body metabolisms will begin occurring in your body, after years of no activity; due to the magnesium deficiency in your diet all these years. Vitamin supplementation is not a gimmick. It's an essential requirement for your health, due to our parched, lifeless, hallow food supply. Just ask yourself WHERE are you getting your daily supply of magnesium in your food? Yea, I know. You can't tell me or yourself!

Now the way you can almost always determine for yourself whether you have kidney disease or whether you have calcium kidney stones or uric acid stones is by doing this:

You almost always notice any kidney problems by the back ache you will get in your lower back. It's not pain. It's aching as though you are just having lower back muscle problems. If you have kidney disease or calcium kidney stones, your lower back will ache almost all the time, BUT, you won't have sharp pains. If your back pain includes sharp pains frequently, then you most likely have uric acid stones. But before I tell you the cure for uric acid kidney stones, I need to explain what to do to determine if your problem is developing chronic kidney disease or calcium kidney stones. Determining this is quite simple, but takes time.

Merely follow my previous instructions to dissolve any calcium kidney stones. And if you do not improve, or a diagnostic test shows your stones still exist, after 6-8 weeks of taking the magnesium and antioxidants, then you have chronic kidney disease. But my strongest advice is to do this, AND, start eliminating the saturation of poisons in our food, drinks and water supplies to speed your cure and healing along, as well as significantly improving your overall health. Use Chapters 5, 6 and 7 for guiding you in eliminating the saturation of poisons in our food, drinks and water supplies; most of which we all pretend are food!

Uric Acid kidney stones – You most likely have uric acid stones from too much uric acid formation from consuming high fructose corn syrup. These stones cannot be cured the same way calcium based kidney stones are cured. To cure uric acid stones drink baking soda and water. You must read food and drink labels and avoid high fructose corn syrup; especially in liquid forms such as soda pops and fruit juice too. Doing so will decrease your body's production of uric acid. The other part of the cure for uric acid stones is to drink lots of pure water to dissolve and flush these stones out of your body. The suggested amount of water is

1 ounce for every 2 pounds of body weight daily. Your kidneys love water. But it needs to be filtered to remove the harmful chlorine and fluoride in the water. Add pH drops or baking soda too.

A carbon water filter only filters out about 90% of the chlorine and nothing else. So that's why you need a fluoride water filter at least. A reverse osmosis is better and filters all your water in your home. Using either of these water filters takes all the taste out of your water that you taste in tap water. The chemicals are bitter and acidic. So by removing chlorine and fluoride, the bitter acidic taste is gone. And your water is alkaline. The easiest way to increase the alkalinity of your water is to add baking soda or pH drops to your drinking water every day. This raises the pH to around 7.5-8.0 and above.

Flushing your kidneys with this highly alkaline water will neutralize acid and slowly transform your body's acidic state back into the normal alkaline state your body is suppose to be in. Your body became acidic over time as you consumed more and more animal products, sugar and chlorinated water. And the highly alkaline water reverses that disease ripe acidic environment inside your body. Chlorine destroys the oxygen in every cell it comes into contact with and kills the beneficial bacteria in your stomach and intestines.

One side effect of the highly alkaline water will be weight loss. As the highly alkaline water neutralizes acid in your body, your kidneys will remove all that water it retained to dilute that acid, as a natural defense to that acid. That is how you lose the weight.

But if none of this causes your lower back ache to go away, you most likely have chronic kidney disease. If so, you will want to read on for the information that will help you and most likely cure you. You can contact Dr. David Moskowitz to participate in his drug treatments to put your kidney disease in check; as I will talk about in Chapter 3. But before I get to the cure and how to avoid dialysis, let me tell you what the doctors did to determine if I had kidney stones.

Well actually they did nothing. But what they wanted me to do and insisted I do was, get some CAT scans of my kidney area at St. Bernard's hospital. When the doctor told me this I said "Why? There's no way I could have kidney stones because I take magnesium." Him and the nurse looked at me like what the heck is he talking about. (Sad, but true, since it's proven medical science.) I asked the employees who scheduled these tests about how much it would cost. No one could tell me. Even St. Bernard's couldn't tell them either until a day later. The cost was $1100. So there was no way I was paying cash for tests that expensive that contradict scientific facts. So I didn't take the CAT scans. Didn't throw away $1100 on unneeded tests.

No. I stuck with proven science instead of trusting the doctor's word that I needed those tests. I didn't have kidney stones and have never had kidney stones. I did have bladder stones in the mid-1990s. And after 4 immensely excruciatingly painful bladder stone attacks, I stopped my fourth bladder stone attack within an hour by talking 2 400mg magnesium oxide tablets. I take magnesium 3 or 4 times a week every week, and haven't had another bladder stone since then, 1996. This was the first time I cured myself of what doctors call "chronic, incurable disease".

It doesn't matter if you have kidney stones, chronic kidney disease or any chronic disease. Doing what Chapters 5, 6 & 7 tell you to do will significantly improve your health and most likely cure you of your chronic diseases. Chronic kidney disease is the deadliest disease, since 100% with chronic kidney disease die from it. Most develop diabetes and die from that. Some develop heart disease. And at some time, most of the rest will go on dialysis, while a small number will receive kidney transplants. Around 20,000 kidney transplants are performed in the United States each year. The waiting list for a kidney has 93,000 people on it, and expands each year by 3000-4000 people.

Now an extremely important thing you should do is use an inexpensive, common substance. It's almost silly what this substance is. It reverses the acidic condition that allowed your kidney disease to survive and thrive in your body. Chronic disease can NOT, I repeat, can NOT live in an alkaline environment. And this common item is none other than baking soda, sodium bicarbonate; also called meetha soda. Diseased cells are also more acidic than the diseased cells in the body.

Baking soda is pH 14, and when mixed with water makes the entire glass of water become a pH of 8.0-8-5. It can be more if you use a carbon water filter, and slightly higher if you use an osmosis system or fluoride filter. Merely mixing 1/2 tea spoon in 4-6 ounces of water and drinking twice daily, before bed and when you awake, will serve as the foundation for your near certain cure.

And don't be fooled by the medical profession. They use sodium bicarbonate to keep chemotherapy patients from dying from the toxicity of their chemical drugs; and for clinical acidosis in patients. It's a vile story about why they stick with their dangerous expensive chemicals in spite of knowing safe, inexpensive natural medicinal solutions. It's all about greed, and greed with no thought of what is good for you, the patient!

You would be well served to find a book by Dr. Mark Sircus tilted simply "Sodium Bicarbonate – Full Medical Review", 2nd edition; a book I only recently found out about. The near miraculous effects of sodium bicarbonate are explained in Dr. Sircus' book. Baking soda will relieve heartburn instantly. It also cures metabolic acidosis of your kidneys which causes almost all chronic kidney disease; and gets you well on your way to curing yourself of CKD.

You can even brush your teeth with it. Just wet your toothbrush. Shake it off once or twice. Then dip it in a box of baking soda to cover your brush with baking soda. Then brush and slosh the liquid around in your mouth a bit. This will neutralize the acid on your teeth and gums, and stop most tooth pain and lessen the severity of sensitivity to heat and cold. Wherever you need to kill fungus or neutralize an acidic substance, remember to call baking soda to the rescue!

There are so many things baking soda is good for. Some of its uses are that it absorbs radiation, alkalizes the body, absorbs heavy metal, treats colds and the flu, treats insect bites and itchy skin, soothes your feet and is a non-toxic deodorant. You can also use it to clean many things like dishes, floors, furniture, shower curtains, baby clothes and cloth diapers, cars, batteries, combs and brushes, and to clean the dirt and residue off fresh produce; as well as clean your bath tub, tile and sinks. Baking soda can also be used as a facial scrub and body exfoliant, to freshen linens, deodorize stinky feet and make a bath soak.

Although all of those uses are great, the lifesaving value of baking soda is the most important. It absorbs radiation, in case of a nuclear attack or exposure such as chemotherapy. Doctors and hospitals use baking soda to keep cancer patients from dying from chemotherapy. And baking soda reverses the acidic state of your body that made it possible for you to develop chronic disease. So make sure you keep plenty of baking soda around. And make sure to drink ½ teaspoon baking soda with 4-6 ounces of water at least 2x daily, as the start and foundation of curing every disease you have and preventing disease from developing in the first place.

I finally cured my gout after I started drinking baking soda water and adding pH drops to my drinking water. It's all simple science. Gout is caused by Uric acid. Highly alkaline substances like baking soda and pH drops neutralize acid, thus reducing the acidic state of your body. It is acid that causes inflammation in your body. So by neutralizing Uric acid with baking soda water and pH drops, you cure your gout.

We use baking soda to neutralize acids, fungi and molds anywhere we find them. We brush our teeth by wetting our brush and covering the brush with baking soda and brushing. And also brush some on our underarms as deodorant. You can also wet your fingers, dip them in the box of baking soda and rub it on your underarms for the best deodorant. So don't ever do without your baking soda!

The next chapter is about Dr. Moskowitz's drug treatments and how to contact him. I also share some of Dr. Moskowitz's insights and some of my experiences with him. Dr. Moskowitz can help you avoid dialysis, but cannot cure you. But you only have to rely on him like any other doctor to get his help. In the chapters after this next chapter about Dr. Moskowitz, the rest of the book is what you can do to significantly improve your health and most likely cure yourself. And the key word there is YOU! I am going to tell YOU how to cure yourself!

I am going to tell you how I cured myself of chronic kidney disease without any help from doctors, after doctors said I would be dead or on dialysis by late 2008 or early 2009. I started developing kidney disease in August 2005 and was diagnosed with chronic kidney disease in October 2006. My creatinine was 3.1 in December 2006.

I will give you the information to avoid dialysis by participating in Dr. Moskowitz's clinically proven drug treatments. Then I will tell you how you can cure yourself and avoid dialysis by doing what I tell you in Chapters 5, 6 & 7.

3 - How to Avoid Dialysis Through Drug Treatments

The only Doctor I could find that was interested in helping people with chronic kidney disease is Dr. David Moskowitz. He is one of the greatest doctors of our time. Dr. Moskowitz is not like all other doctors of my life time. He doesn't prolong your diseases to maximize his income as all doctors do. Nope. Dr. Moskowitz has worked tirelessly to discover a way to hold kidney disease in check so that you can avoid dialysis.

Although Dr. Moskowitz and I have a doctor-patient relationship, we have also become friends and talk about things beyond your normal doctor-patient relationship. This is true for several reasons. First of all, I had gotten my creatinine down to as low as 2.2 on my own, prior to knowing Dr. Moskowitz. But it would fluctuate up a little from time to time and worry me. But since I began Dr. Moskowitz's drug treatment, my creatinine has stayed no higher than 2.3 and as low as 1.8. So Dr. Moskowitz, and even my current M.D. Dr. Allen, have their own scientific proof that what I did for myself does indeed work. And Dr. Allen and I also has the proof that Dr. Moskowitz's drug treatments work.

It is most certainly the best choice to do what I did and cure yourself, not only of chronic kidney disease, but every chronic disease you have. But that is not the way people do things in this country. You trust corporations and the phony FDA, and that is what is causing the deaths of almost every citizen of the United States. The FDA says the deadly disease producing poisons produced by food and drink corporations are "safe". The thing you have to do is snap out of that insane way of thinking. Poisons are harmful; harmful to your health, but THE main factor in addicting you to their products. I will talk about this later.

But for now, I am just pointing out that it is your own self-destructive ways that are causing almost all sickness and disease. Yes, YOU are making YOU sick! And since rare few ever take responsibility for their own lives in this immoral nation, all rely on doctors.

So the easiest, laziest, thing to do is just pay a doctor to try and fix what you have done to yourself. But there is no Doctor in the country that will do anything to put your kidney disease in check, much less cure you. Doctors have no cures. And that includes my dear friend Dr. David Moskowitz. But what Dr. Moskowitz can and will do for you is help you to avoid dialysis by taking a special dosage of a well-known drug that is usually used to help control blood pressure.

But to do that, you and Dr. Moskowitz will need the cooperation of your family Physician merely supporting the simple goal of you staying off dialysis and not dying. As reasonable as this seems, most or all of you will find that your doctors probably won't be interested. At least that was the biggest obstacle I faced when I was trying to find a doctor who would go along with me being cured or them cooperating with Dr. Moskowitz's drug treatments to avoid dialysis. It took a major effort on my part over a period of at least 5 months to find one doctor who would at least be open to something that could help me avoid dialysis.

And even then, the doctor only agreed to go along at first to see if there was any scientific proof that what Dr. Moskowitz was doing would help. The doctors that first diagnosed me with chronic kidney disease never tried to help me. But when they had their own scientific proof that what I was doing was reversing my chronic kidney disease, they threw me out of their Clinic, Clopton Clinic.

They had absolutely no interest in finding out what I had done to achieve what no doctor had ever achieved. Instead, they sent me certified letters telling me they would no longer be my doctors. There went one of their $100,000 a year dialysis ponies. And that was all they ever cared about. So that's why I advise you to do things my way WHILE you are trying to get the cooperation of a local doctor so that you can get on Dr. Moskowitz's drug treatments.

I gave you all these facts to warn you about how, even though it seems like a very simple matter, doctors have no cures and have no interest in you being cured or getting better. And that turns a simple matter into an impossible situation. This book is about YOU avoiding dialysis and/or curing yourself, or at least greatly improving your health, and adding days, weeks and years to your life.

So, to avoid dialysis you can contact Dr. David Moskowitz to take part in his clinically proven treatments that will put your kidney disease in check within 6-8 weeks. And while you are doing that, you can also cure yourself naturally like I did; using natural methods which cost very little money and usually end up saving you money on groceries. Curing yourself naturally takes time and your efforts, while Dr. Moskowitz's treatments only require you paying a small fee and the cooperation of your family Physician supporting the simple goal of you staying off dialysis and not dying!

Now let me tell you what I know about Dr. David Moskowitz and his words, views and responses on relevant issues and a few questions I asked him.

Dr. David Moskowitz – He Stands Alone!

When I was doing one of my SEARCHES on the INTERNET for avoiding dialysis about mid-2008, one return was for GenoMed. It hadn't been there in previous SEARCHES. The best thing I had found up until the day I found GenoMed was Dr. Mackenzie Walser's book about Avoiding Dialysis called Coping with Kidney Disease: A 12-Step Program to Help You Avoid Dialysis. I bought his book and it was the only outside help I had gotten for my kidneys at that time. Dr. Moskowitz later told me "I had the enormous pleasure of meeting Mackenzie Walser in person about 20 years ago at a small conference on nutrition and the kidney in northern Virginia. He was terrific!" I was glad to hear Dr. Moskowitz's approval of Dr. Walser.

I contacted Dr. Moskowitz the same day I had found GenoMed's web site. I asked him if he could help me and he said he could, but we needed to get started right away since my creatinine was still 2.37 at that time, August 21, 2008. It took me from August 21 until December 8 to find a doctor who would help me get on Dr. Moskowitz's treatment program. But, on December 8, 2008 I started his program. It took me until April 2009, four months, to completely get on Dr. Moskowitz's treatment he said would hold my kidney disease in check.

We exchanged dozens of emails and I paid him $75 a month to be a part of his program. Dr. Moskowitz stuck in there with me while I was trying to get a doctor to go along with his treatment for me. It wasn't his responsibility to do so, but he cared enough to help me get through all the obstacles being hurled at me by the hideous medical profession. He cared about this and helped before I had ever paid him a penny and has continued to be a beloved friend even after I stopped paying him. He has always been thrilled to see me staying off dialysis, and has told me he appreciates any credit I will give him for that.

I was afraid to speak out about what sick jerks doctors are in my opinion, because I was concerned about those facts being disrespectful toward Dr. Moskowitz; just as I have been concerned about my current M.D., Dr. Allen in the same way. But the medical profession has given

Dr. Moskowitz a lot more crap than they have me! Sure my life was on the line, but Dr. Moskowitz's career, reputation and life have been in jeopardy ever since he made serious and significant advances in the prevention of chronic disease and grown in that lifesaving work.

So I asked Dr. Moskowitz about this recently, if any government agencies were doing their job of spreading the word to the Public about his superior outcome clinical trials. Dr. Moskowitz's reply was "Absolutely not. The Kidney Institute of the NIH (NIDDK) says it can't understand the paper I published. Yet they haven't asked me to explain it to them. The CDC has been completely unhelpful, refusing to answer my emails and phone calls."

As part of that question I also asked Dr. Moskowitz about the VA taking over 1000 of his patients off his treatment program for avoiding dialysis and he added "They just lowered the dose of prescribed medication each day. The prescribed drug was on the formulary, so there was no reason to change the medication. Sure enough, all my patients whose creatinines were stable or even going down started doing worse within a month or two, their creatinines started going up again. I was only able to watch for 6 months before the VA took away my computer privileges and fired me. I called my trial an "inadvertent cross-over design."

Dr. Moskowitz made his feelings about his experiences with the government and medical profession even clearer saying "If my boss at the VA had responded appropriately in 1996 and been open-minded enough to see the outcomes of my 1000 patients, instead of dismissing my data from the previous 2 years as merely "anecdotal" and refusing even to look at it, we'd live in a different world. For one thing, it would already be dialysis-free. I reckon a million Americans would have been kept off the dialysis machine and remained alive, at a savings of half a trillion dollars. Not to mention the savings in life and treasure in the rest of the world."

"Everybody in a position to help, refused to. Everybody receiving a salary to promote public health chose instead not to say a word. I am absolutely flabbergasted at the wholesale failure of our public health institutions. It's as if we live in an anti-world where everything is the opposite of what it's supposed to be. No wonder the public is busy trying alternative medicine! They must sense at some deep level that mainstream medicine is doing everything it can to keep their disease around and keep getting rich from it. The rot is much greater than I ever thought."

Dr. Moskowitz' then concluded saying "I just think about how health care has changed. In the early 1950s, there was a hunger to defeat disease. TB fell, polio fell and rheumatic fever had just fallen in the late 1940s with the introduction of penicillin. I was taught that medicine was still like that, when I was in Med school in the late 1970s. But managed care and the fear of malpractice have crippled American medicine. Now medicine is anti-intellectual, risk-averse, and celebrates the status quo. For a variety of reasons, health care no longer does any clinically meaningful research. We're told that American medicine is the best in the world, when people are still practicing the way we did in the 1970s and early 80s. Medicine has become frozen in time."

I had told Dr. Moskowitz I was asking these questions for my book and that I didn't want to appear to be dragging him into my realization about the entire medical profession being interested ONLY in prolonging disease to maximize their income.

The help I have gotten from Dr. Moskowitz and his scientifically proven treatment is a major factor in me avoiding dialysis for years. Yes I had already gotten my creatinine down to 2.2 before I even heard of Dr. Moskowitz. But my creatinine had never gone down to 1.8 before! My creatinine was 2.37 when I started Dr. Moskowitz's program. And my creatinine has stayed lower than 2.37 the 2 ½ years I've been on his treatment, averaging 2.1 and has gone down to 1.9 twice and is now 1.8. I had run out of ideas as to how to get my creatinine to go any lower when I first talked to Dr. Moskowitz. So there's no way I will agree to stop his drug treatment. To refresh my memory on who Dr. Moskowitz can actually help, I asked him a few questions to clarify this in order to help others.

As for all the other patients who have used Dr. Moskowitz's treatment for chronic kidney disease he says - "My very first patient, I remember, was a black man with high blood pressure and a creatinine of 3.1. I started him on a high-dose of a prescription drug the month before. When I saw him back the next month, his creatinine should have increased on its own to 3.3 or so. But it was 2.8. It kept going down, but the VA took him away from me before his creatinine got below 2. And how have his patients done?

"Since 1994, of all my patients with a creatinine around 2 or less, I

haven't had one go on dialysis, unless they had a high creatinine already. In all, I'd say about 1300 patients so far" says Dr. Moskowitz.

So when does a patient need to start your treatment? 2.3 Or what? I asked him. Dr. Moskowitz replied saying "Before it reaches 3.5 for sure. The lower it is when they first contact me, the lower it will remain. Above 3.5, I could still try to slow down their kidney failure, but we may not get anywhere. The higher the creatinine, the less hope I have, but I'd be willing to try to help anyone. Once on dialysis, though, I'm afraid it's hopeless. Terry, thanks for trusting me enough to let me try to help you. It takes a huge amount of courage to try something new, something that none of your doctors tell you could work."

Understanding how Dr. Moskowitz's treatment works, I asked him "Are you a genetic scientist?" But Dr. Moskowitz says "I'd call my field genomic epidemiology rather than genetics." I know how his treatment neutralizes the part of the gene that promotes my kidney disease. And with all the DNA altering and gene mutating poisons in our nation's food, drinks and water supplies, work such as Dr. Moskowitz is doing must be continued and expanded.

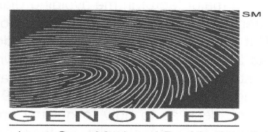

To find out more about GenoMed and Dr. Moskowitz's treatments for chronic diseases, go to the GenoMed web site. - www.GenoMed.com

4 - How to Cure Kidney Disease Naturally, Without Doctors

If you want to cure yourself or at least significantly improve your health, then I can tell you how to do that. That's what I had to do for myself to save my own life, after doctors said I would be dead or on dialysis by 2008. And even when you are on dialysis, it's almost like already being dead. I had one friend for sure that was just in his 30's when he started dialysis. He didn't last but 3 or 4 years after he started dialysis. And his quality of life was real bad too. So I was almost terrified as I looked to the future and knew I would soon be dead or on dialysis.

But no matter who I talked to, I never found any hope of anyone getting better once they had chronic kidney disease. I searched and searched the INTERNET for cures for kidney disease and avoiding dialysis and similar search strings, from the day doctors told me I had chronic kidney disease. But I couldn't find anything. About the only help I found was a book by Dr. Mackenzie Walser called Coping with Kidney Disease: A 12-Step Program to Help You Avoid Dialysis.

Dr. Walser's book detailed his clinical research with his patients in testing his variation of a zero protein diet used by the British to successfully delay dialysis. Dr. Walser created a low protein diet to delay dialysis. The best this could do was to achieve what is called arrested progression. This means the progression of your chronic kidney disease has been arrested, stopped. But Dr. Walser states this is not remission. Remission is where you reverse the kidney disease, and your kidneys improve for longer than a few months or you cure your kidney disease. Well, I know Dr. Walser would be thrilled to know what I achieved. I consider myself cured of chronic kidney disease.

But what are the details of that "cure"? First of all, I don't have any symptoms of chronic kidney disease any more. At first, my blood pressure was 240/140. I pissed blood and blood clots. I was excruciatingly tense and tight all over my body from low Potassium. I spent at least 2/3 of every day trying to piss, but barely did. I couldn't sleep, and only slept maybe 2 hours a night for weeks.

Then once I begin to get lab test results, my above normal results were Creatinine at 2.9 and my BUN was 30. I was also leaking protein into my urine. And my Potassium was below normal at 2.9. My EKG showed that I had an enlarged heart and I had dozens of bruises all over my body where blood vessels had popped from the 240/140 blood pressure. And when my next lab results came back, they showed I was getting worse! My Creatinine continued to climb to 3.1. My BUN jumped to 44. And my Potassium jumped from 2.9 to 5.7. Normal for those 3 are 1.5, 8-24 and a 3.5 - 5.0 range for Potassium.

But since I began doing the things I will share with you in Chapters 5, 6 and 7, my Creatinine has been as low as 1.8. My Potassium has been normal the whole time. And everything else in my blood serum lab tests have been normal. My EKGs also changed and the results were good, then very good. I never have those attacks of shortness of breath either, that are caused by an enlarged heart. My doctor began treating me as though I am not a kidney patient. He has his own scientific proof of what I have done.

So whether you agree that I have indeed cured myself, I know you can all agree that I sure live in the threshold of being cured. And I have been there since the middle of 2007; even though I didn't realize I had actually succeeded in reversing my chronic kidney disease until I had sustained that remission for a few years.

In 2009 I began to dismiss dialysis and Death as my only future and began to take my life back and start living again. In 2010, I was continuing to take my life back. And in 2011, I began to be a useful, productive person again. I wrote my first two books in 2011. And became more and more active, with the fear of dialysis and death becoming more and more just a fading memory.

Dialysis is not the solution you want. It is very hard on you. It's a fact that 1 out of every 5 people who go on dialysis, take themselves off of dialysis; as death is a better choice than dialysis to that 20%. I for one, celebrate every day about how I am still alive and dialysis free, here in 2012, seven years after my chronic kidney disease first began to develop and progress. My CKD began in August 2005. It took me almost 20 months after it began, to begin to arrest my kidney disease. And that would continue to this very moment.

So HOW did I manage to do what no doctors have ever done, and do so without any real help from doctors?

That is what I will be explaining now, and giving you the information you need to empower yourself to cure yourself or at least significantly improving your health, and extending your life by days, weeks and most likely for years. And you can do what I did, even if you participate in Dr.

Moskowitz's drug treatments to avoid dialysis, and even WHILE you let your doctors hold your hand and lead you to your grave as they prolong your illness to maximize their income.

You WILL become the doctors' $100,000 a year dialysis pony unless you contact Dr. Moskowitz, or do what I did, OR BOTH!

So here we go with my way of reversing chronic kidney disease and avoiding dialysis naturally. What you have to do is change your diet. It's the saturation of poisons in our food, drinks and water supplies that are making us all sick to the point that over 130,000,000 Americans have at least one chronic disease. All disease is caused by poisons, toxins, chemicals; except for the 20% caused by germs and viruses. Your kidneys are the main organ for removing toxins from your body. And as you overload your kidneys with poisons, those poisons back up in your kidneys and began to saturate your kidneys with those poisons. Your kidneys begin to turn to mush, then your kidney disease becomes noticeable. But by then, it's too late.

When this happened to me, I not only had to deal with being sick, I had to figure out something that might help my kidneys get better. The doctors sure did nothing for my kidneys; even though I asked them to help my kidneys every time I went to the doctor! They even began to think I was crazy because I kept telling them I wanted to be cured. I didn't realize it while it was happening. I read it on my medical records later. I'm dying and they won't help! So what are you going to do?

Do everything this book says to do in Chapters 5, 6 and 7. Chapter 5 is called Poisons in Your Water. I explain things about the water we drink; including bottled water. To sum the chapter up, simply forget about bottled water. PERIOD. And get a shower filter and a drinking water filter; preferably a fluoride filter. That's because a fluoride filter removes everything but the water at a rate of about 99%.

A shower filter is a special hot water filter that eliminates at least 90% of the chlorine in your shower water. Doing that cures dandruff and dry itchy red spots caused by the chlorine destroying the oils in our scalp and skin; and kills the oxygen in every cell it comes into contact with. Without a shower filter, you are absorbing chlorine and fluoride through every pore on your body, while breathing chlorine gas in the steam of the hot shower water. So this is a major source of poisons for everyone. And that makes a shower filter a MUST for kidney patients.

Chapter 6 talks about the saturation of poisons in our drinks, like sodas, fruit juices and milk. Beware of how sad these facts are. It's rare to find any drink product at the grocery store that is NOT saturated with poisons. I do explain some alternatives which you can drink, that aren't highly poisonous. But it pretty much comes down to Stevia sweetened tea, 2% or Skim milk and organic milk and a new soda, like 7-UP, called Sierra Mist.

Then in Chapter 7, I give you the information to guide you in greatly reducing and eliminating almost all poisons from your food supply. It includes detailed information about sugars and also about the fraudulent labeling terms most food corporations use to try and trick you into buying their "healthy" products! You can't allow yourself to be fooled by terms like "Natural, All Natural, Low Fat, Reduced Fat, Low Calorie, 100% Juice and other big fat lies. And there is no worse poison than high fructose corn syrup. It was high fructose corn syrup in the sodas and fruit juices I drank daily for about 5 years that are responsible for my kidney failure.

Now, before I end this chapter so you can get on to the information that saved my life and reversed my chronic kidney disease, I need to explain some rules, laws, principles that my methods are founded on. If you take time to learn these scientific principles, you will value my methods much better and speed your cure along. It is these principles that my methods are founded on. One of those principles is about how your body can heal itself.

You have cut yourself before, right? Do you still have that cut? No. It healed on its own. And did you know that your liver can grow new cells. Say, if you had part of your liver removed, it grows back. So I am very confident in our bodies' ability to heal us of anything we do to ourselves, except for serious blunt trauma or the likes. But you have to know how to make your body work to heal you better if you are going to cure yourself of chronic disease. The way to do that is to fast.

It is not necessary to fast for days. By simply eating your last meal around 6 PM, then not eating again until between 6 and 10 AM the next day, will do a lot for you; especially if you make it a habit. Fasting was the foundation of the medical practices of Hippocrates, the Father of Medicine. What fasting does is to relieve the body of the most energy consuming bodily task of digesting food. Once your body ceases to digest food, your body then uses that energy to repair damaged cells in our bodies. And when you are sick, your body needs to use as much energy as possible to repair damaged cells and remove toxins, as it possibly can. And the less poisons you put into your body, the less energy your body has to use to remove those toxins. A good example is when you drink a soda pop.

People fool themselves by thinking that soda pop gives them a welcome energy boost! But it's no energy boost! What really happens is this: You begin drinking that sugar soaked soda in liquid form with that DNA altering sodium benzoate and that 3.0 acidic carbonated water and your body goes into instant shock as it tries to defend itself against all that poison. This instant elevated activity the body goes into to remove these poisons is what we falsely tell ourselves is just an energy boost. And it takes your body up to 6 hours to remove the poisons in a 12 ounce soda pop. That cripples your immune system. And by drinking a 12 ounce soda every 6 hours, you in effect, nullify your immune system.

So, your body only has so much energy. It uses most of its energy to digest food. It uses the rest of its energy to remove toxins and repair damaged cells. So you have to learn how to make your body use more and more of its energy to repair damaged cells to heal and cure you. The easiest way to do that is to fast as often as possible and cut down on the amount of food you eat. Using chapters 5, 6 and 7 to reduce the amount of poisons you consume in your food, drinks and water will relieve your body of having to use so much energy to remove toxins from your body. Doing this and fasting allows your body to use most of its energy to repair damaged cells, which eventually results in you being cured.

You also have to understand that you need to eat as healthy a diet and drinks as you can. I mean, why drink a soda or fruit juice when you could drink something that your body doesn't have to work so hard to remove all the poisons in that soda or juice. You could drink fruit smoothies made with raw fruits. That would be almost 100% good for your body. Those live fruits and vegetables have enzymes that pump life into your body. And your body doesn't work to remove that live produce. Your body uses most of that live produce. And if you juice that produce, it's easier for your body to digest than solid food.

It takes far less energy to digest that produce if you run them through a good juice making machine. But even if you don't juice or don't do it often, you can still try to eat as much raw fruits and vegetables as you possibly can. As a matter of fact, if you just those water filters and just follow what I call The Perfect Diet, you can cure yourself or significantly improve your health without having to learn how to read food labels and avoid the masses of products that are saturated with poisons; most of which we pretend are food. So what do I mean by The Perfect Diet? The Perfect Diet is the best diet to be on. But since it is a far cry from the "American diet", you may do best by using Chapters 6 & 7 to clean up your current diet that caused your diseases in the first place.

The Perfect Diet....

What do I mean by The Perfect Diet? If I could eat the most healthy diet of food and drinks, what would that diet consist of? Right off you would say eat fresh fruits and vegetables ONLY and drink pure water The problem you would have is that there are poisons inside all produce in this country. So you would have to buy all Organic; which is not possible without restricting your diet even further. You could grow all the produce yourself, or hire someone to do it for you, if you can afford to. So, the perfect diet is not practical in this country and the life styles we live in this country.

You could grow all your own food organically and drink pure water. But as soon as you are forced to send your children to school, they'll gag them with poison saturated food. But the Perfect Diet would be to grow all your food organically and drink pure water. You can grow peaches, figs, apples, grapes, Kiwi, Strawberries and all kinds of fruits to go along with your organic vegetables. Stick to drinking pure water, and you're on the Perfect Diet! But since we all know how impractical this is, we have to present an idea or ideas that are achievable for most people. So how do we come close to having the Perfect Diet, living in this country?

The obvious is just buy produce from the grocery store and wash it extra good, and make as much of that produce as you can, Organic produce. Then buy Organic 2% milk. Eat lots and lots of brown rice. Drink Lipton tea sweetened with Stevia. Buy only whole fish or fillets. No breading. Bake your own whole grain breads and don't add the sick crap to them, like vegetable oils, margarine, white flour and white granulated sugar.

Buy frozen produce when fresh is not available. Never buy canned. And use raw honey anywhere you want and as much as you want. Drink lots of pure Noni, Goji and Mangosteen juice or Goji berries. Add dried fruits and nuts to your diet. And even adding all these things beyond the ultimate Perfect Diet, you still have a near perfect diet.

And that's The Perfect Diet! But for most of you, you will want to read on and use Chapters 6 & 7 as a guide from now on to avoid those poisons that saturate our entire food and drinks supplies.

You can contact Dr. Moskowitz if your Creatinine is 3.9 or less. But regardless of what your Creatinine is, you can go on The Perfect Diet or clean up your own current poison saturated diet. And if your Creatinine is above 3.9, all you can do is go on The Perfect Diet or clean up your current diet. And one of the most important parts of doing that, is to reduce the amount of protein you eat. Fact is, too much protein is a cause of some kidney disease and failure.

So keep the principles in mind at all times that I just discussed in this chapter, while you change to The Perfect Diet or choose to clean up your current diet by using Chapters 6 and 7 as your guide. Your body is 80% water. Drinking 1 ounce of water per 2 pounds of body weight daily helps clean out your body and flush large amounts of toxins out through your urine.

So I begin with **Poisons in Your Water.**

5 -Poisons in Your Water

It is very important that I talk to you about the poisons in your water first. The first city to provide chlorinated water in the US was Jersey City in 1908. At least 70% of the US population gets their water from systems relying on chlorine; although 90% of the water systems in the US rely on chlorination in one form or the other. Chlorine was first used in water supplies to stop typhoid. Researchers claim this actually worked, and have presented proof that chlorine kills other water borne diseases. I don't doubt any of this. As a matter of fact, if it wasn't for the chlorine in your water you would get sick shortly after drinking water in city water systems.

So I agree that the chlorine needs to be in the water to kill germs. But guess what? Chlorine kills bacteria. Oh, you already knew that! But what rare few ever realize is that chlorine keeps right on being itself and kills bacteria once it's inside your body. And that is what no one is talking about. Your water supplier sure doesn't want to talk about it either.

I called our water supplier called CW&L. The Manager of CW&L certainly admitted to the chlorine and fluoride they put in our water. But he refused to agree to warn the Public about the dangers and adverse consequences of drinking and showering in their chlorinated water. I told him point blank "You need to take the fluoride out of the water. It should never have been put in our water."

As he pretended to defend his position in favor of the poisons, he pointed out how beneficial fluoride is in preventing a few cavities. What he didn't want to talk about is what fluoride has to do with safe drinking water or the many cases of brittle bones, chromosome damage and other conditions known to be caused by fluoride ingestion. The fluoride in drinking water has absolutely no benefit beyond this claim about preventing cavities.

But hey, we could add vitamin C to the water. It's good for you. Or add other things that are good for us. That is, if you don't care about clean water! Whoops! You mean CW&L has lost touch with reality and no longer realizes that our water supply is NOT the place to be adding chemicals or anything else. Water is H2O, NOT H2O+chlorine+fluoride! I want WATER, H2O! But I can't get it. So I gotta give it to myself by getting a fluoride water filter. It would be so easy IF CW&L would stop being CWL&Dental and start being CW&L again! But they refuse. So I gotta keep using a fluoride water filter. No problem, except for the $110 to buy a fluoride water filter.

But even though chlorine and fluoride cause a host of diseases, the most significant damage that immediately affects everyone who drinks it is how chlorine kills the beneficial bacteria in your stomach and intestines. Remember, I already pointed out that chlorine is in your water to kill bacteria! And **chlorine keeps right on killing bacteria once it's inside your body!** Is this good? NO. That beneficial bacteria in your stomach and intestines is required to sustain your life.

As these bacteria, flora, are killed your body digests less of your food. This issue is so important that I want you to read some technical facts about this bacteria, gut flora. So I am including what Wikipedia says about this, even though most of you can just SEARCH Wikipedia for "gut flora". Here's exactly what Wikipedia states:

Gut flora consists of microorganisms that live in the digestive tracts of animals and is the largest reservoir of human flora. Gut (the adjective) is synonymous with intestinal, and flora with microbiota and microflora. The human body, consisting of about 100 trillion cells, carries about ten times as many microorganisms in the intestines. The metabolic activities performed by these bacteria resemble those of an organ, leading some to liken gut bacteria to a "forgotten" organ. It is estimated that these gut flora have around 100 times as many genes in aggregate as there are in the human genome. Bacteria make up most of the flora in the colon and up to 60% of the dry mass of feces. Somewhere between 300 and 1000 different species live in the gut, with most estimates at about 500. However, it is probable that 99% of the bacteria come from about 30 or 40 species. Fungi and protozoa also make up a part of the gut flora, but little is known about their activities.

Research suggests that the relationship between gut flora and humans is not merely a non-harmful coexistence, but rather a symbiotic relationship. Though people can survive without gut flora, the microorganisms perform a host of useful functions, such as fermenting unused energy substrates, training the immune system, preventing growth of harmful, pathogenic bacteria, regulating the development of the gut, producing vitamins for the host (such as biotin and vitamin K), and producing hormones to direct the host to store fats. However, in certain conditions, some species are thought to be capable of causing disease by producing infection or increasing cancer risk for the host.

Now that you have some in depth information about the bacteria, flora, in your stomach and intestines and its tremendous importance, now I'll tell you how killing this bacteria, by drinking chlorinated water, affects you and your health. The most common condition affects how much you eat. Almost all of us drink chlorinated water our entire childhood lives.

After 18 years of doing this you have significantly reduced the amount of good bacteria in your stomach and intestines. As a result, you eat a good meal, but you are hungry again within an hour and a half to two hours later. Why? Because you are mistaking the barren feeling in your stomach as hunger pains. So you eat food to feel something in your stomach.

Eating sugary foods, drinking sugary drinks and eating white flour aggravates and burns your stomach and intestines making this empty barren feeling even worse! Then heartburn begins as a further sign of this damage to your stomach and intestines. Then your intestines begin to bleed and you bleed out your bunghole, or rectum for you technically minded people.

Your doctor calls this bleeding ulcers, but can't really do a thing for you; although doctors do trick people into having surgery to correct this. Uh, cough, gag, stumble, puke! But is there any condition that doctors do NOT claim you need surgery for?!?

Yes you need surgery so doctors can make big bucks off your disease and suffering. But for you to be cured of bleeding ulcers, you're gonna need to learn what I am telling you. I wish I could charge a small percentage of the huge amounts of money the information in this book saves you, compared to what the medical industry charges you to never cure you, but treat and drug your diseases and medical conditions. I could hire you as my servants! LOL Sorry. I know how serious this is, but the helpless corrupt medical profession makes me laugh.

What can I do to replenish this good bacteria killed by chlorine? There are several things you can do. You can take probiotics. That's what I did. Believe me. I didn't know much of anything when I was learning the things I talk about in this book. So I used myself as a guinea pig to experiment and test these things. Make sure you read chapter 8 where I explain how I came to know and prove that the things I am talking about are true and really work. Don't let the title of the chapter mislead you. That chapter is me telling my story about how I came to learn what is in this book, and how I was forced to save my own life or be on dialysis by 2008 or dead by 2009 as the doctors insisted.

I started taking probiotics. I started out just taking some Lactobacillus acidophilus and B. Lactis, also known as Acidophilus complex. But once I started taking Dr. Ohirra's Probiotics 12 Plus I started noticing some improvement. I wasn't hungry shortly after eating and my stomach felt much better. I am still taking Dr. Ohirra's Probiotics from time to time and take the Acidophilus complex daily, usually more than once a day with meals. Buy the Acidophilus with the most active cultures. I use the one with 1 billion live organisms per capsule.

Capsules are much easier to digest and therefore provide the greatest benefit compared to caplets or tablets. Acidophilus is the easiest pro-biotic to find. It's one of two bacteria usually found in yogurt. Probiotics with 10-12 different bacteria or more are a little harder to find, but provide the greatest health benefits; especially a natural probiotics product such as Dr. Ohhira's Probiotics.

Eating fresh, raw fruits and vegetables aid in the production of beneficial bacteria in your stomach and intestines too. The enzymes in raw fruits and vegetables are the key to this aid, and do so many other beneficial things to improve your health and heal your body. So eat as much fresh, raw fruits and vegetables as you can.

There are lots of books explaining the endless health benefits of fresh fruits and vegetables, so I will not go into this in depth. Fresh fruits and vegetables provide generous amounts of fiber to protect your stomach and intestines, aid in digestion, nourish and heal damaged cells and promote regular bowel movements.

People whose diets are lacking in fresh fruits and vegetables and fiber rarely have bowel movements every day. Fact is, you should have a bowel movement not too long after each meal. Most of you will say that's crazy. No one has a bowel movement after each meal or most meals! But what I say to you is this. It's NOT crazy either. Want some proof? Oki dokey people! Any of you ever have children? Ah ha!

You only changing poopy diapers ONCE each day! I think NOT! When you are born and a baby, your stomach and intestines are healthy. You know, before you start killing your insides with chlorinated water, antibiotics, sugars and more. So you poop after each meal usually. But as you bombard your intestines with all these poisons, your body goes to work trying to protect itself against all these poisons. As a result, your intestines get coated with mucus. Mucus looks like snot and boogers mixed together; which you see in your poop quite often. Once this mucus coats your intestines, your intestines have a harder and harder time of digesting and absorbing nutrients.

In addition, you start developing pockets in your intestines which your poop begins to move into. Some people have 5-10 pounds of poop stuck in these pockets in your intestines; which stay in your intestines rotting for years, causing even more discomfort and health problems.

Doing a colon cleanse will do a lot in solving this problem. There are lots of different colon cleanses on the market. Most of them aren't very good. But I have tried a few of them. The best ones I have found are called Colonix and Almighty Cleanse. But here's a link you can go to and read about the top colon cleansers and make your own choice. www.detoxreviews.com If you do any internal cleanses, make sure you do a colon cleanse first. That way, if you did a liver cleanse, kidney cleanse or any other internal cleanse you won't cause yourself problems by overloading your intestines with poisons.

So cleanse your colon, then do other cleanses to be safe and as effective as possible. Although the cause of Elvis Presley's death was ruled as a heart attack, his doctors had treated Elvis for chronic constipation for over a decade before his death, and now believe Elvis's death was actually caused by chronic constipation.

Elvis' autopsy revealed that Elvis' digestive system was a real mess when he died and that Elvis would've have lived longer if he had a colostomy. I know that doing a colon cleanse certainly helped me. The proof was how it made me feel better and lighter inside and by looking at my own poop when I was doing colon cleanses. I go by results, not the price of the product or the sales pitch and advertisements about the product.

I want to point out to you right now that it was necessary for me to talk about the poisons in your water first, before I talked about anything else for a very good reason. As you read this book there are many things I recommend that you put into your body. But these vitamins, herbs, foods and other items have to be digested properly. So the more beneficial bacteria you have in your stomach and intestines, the better you digest these items and thus, the more you benefit from taking them.

In some people these vitamins, herbs and foods may seem to do you very little good if the beneficial bacteria in your stomach and intestines is greatly depleted. So, for these vitamins, herbs and foods to do you more good and benefit you more greatly you will need to take probiotics as the first thing to do. Then you will get the greatest benefits from taking supplements, herbs and healthy foods in the most cost effective and efficient manner.

About the most important thing you can do about the poisons in your water is to get some type of water filter. You need one for your drinking and cooking water and one for your shower. Yes, you need a shower filter. But first let's look at the solution for needing a water filter. You can buy inexpensive faucet end carbon water filters. Years ago, we bought a Water Pik faucet end filter. It does a lot of good for about $20. You can buy easily replaceable carbon filter cartridges for about $5 each or a 4 pack for around $16.

We got ours at Lowe's back in the 80's and used it till we got a cylinder shaped counter top carbon water filter from HSN. These filters are worth the money if that is all you can afford or care to invest at first. What you really need is a fluoride filter. A carbon filter only filters out about 90% of the chlorine, some dirt and other impurities, but not a speck of fluoride. Fluoride is a smaller particle and requires a better filter to eliminate it.

Fluoride filters – Fluoride filters are my filter of choice. Sure, I'd like to have a whole house osmosis filtration system, but the fluoride water filter we use is really great. The chlorine and fluoride give tap water a bitter taste which you get use to after drinking it that way for years. But I always do a little test to show people the difference between water and chlorinated, fluoridated water.

I take two identical glasses. Pour chlorinated, fluoridated water in one glass and pure water from our fluoride water filter in the other glass, and ask them to tell me if they can tell any difference and which one they like the best. 100% of the people so far always say the water that came from the fluoride water filter is the best and know which is which. I also ask them "What does the water from the fluoride filter taste like?" Their answer "Nothing" or "It doesn't have any taste". I tell them "Right, because it's WATER!"

When we first got our fluoride water filter, my wife and I would giggle every time after drinking some water. Hey, don't bash us! hehe We couldn't help it. Every drink of water going down our throats is pure and tasteless! Neither of us had ever had that experience. We felt highly privileged to be drinking water so pure. We even thought it was stupid that we felt that way about a water filter! Problem is, we are worse about it now than we were at the first. I love that pure water. You can drink all you want and it does absolutely no harm, and does so much good for your body and your health.

Having pure water from our fluoride water filter may have been the #1 factor in saving my life or at least sparing my life for years so far. Even doctors will tell you that your kidneys love water. And the fact that I was diagnosed with chronic kidney disease a few months earlier made pure water become the thing I began to consume the most.

You need one ounce of water for every two pounds of body weight daily. For me that's around three quarts daily. I never drank that much water in my life, and the older I got the less water I drank. Fortunately for me, the past 30 years I've been drinking filtered water. I sometimes think about how much chlorine I have NOT consumed and the internal damage that comes with drinking tap water.

Your body has to filter out every bit of that chlorine and fluoride, and almost all of that work is handled by your kidneys. Once your kidneys get saturated with so much poison that they can't remove all of it from your body as quickly as you pour and stuff those poisons down your throat, your kidneys will begin to fail. I'll tell you how that happened to me in Chapter 8.

What about a shower filter? I believe a shower filter is at least as important as having a filter on your drinking and cooking water. I never thought about having a shower filter my whole life and honestly had never heard of such a thing. I didn't know anything about shower filters until after I bought one. Now, sometimes I get to thinking a shower filter is more important than a filter for drinking and cooking water; which bolsters my opinion that you need both and should see them both as necessities.

The main reason I believe this is because **you soak up about ten times as much chlorine and fluoride in the shower as you generally do through drinking and cooking water.** Water causes the pores in your skin to expand; which allows greater absorption into your body and bloodstream.

After we got our shower filter I could tell right off that the water coming out of the shower filter no longer had that chemical chlorine smell. I even got a large glass of tap water to sniff in the shower; which I then sniffed the water coming out of the shower filter. The tap water had that familiar chlorine smell, and the filtered shower water had no smell. Then I just left it to hopefully do what I bought it for.

A few weeks later my wife and I both got a good surprise. We have had burning itchy places on our bodies over the years. We blamed cold weather, taking too many showers and maybe a few other things, but never got rid of those itchy red places.

When I looked back soon after this, I realized while in the shower that those red itchy places were the exact places where the most shower water hits my body. Our good surprise was that we no longer had those red itchy places just 3 weeks after installing our shower filter! I got on the INTERNET to SEARCH for something to explain our good surprise.

As it turns out, the chlorine in tap water destroys the oils in your skin and… YOUR HAIR! Got dandruff! I bet you do after burn drying your scalp with chlorinated water! I repeat. **The chlorine in your shower water dries out your skin, scalp and hair by destroying the oils in your skin, scalp and hair!**

Don't calm down yet! LOL Here's what could be the worst part. (I say this very sincerely and make the following comparison to save lives, and for this reason, the following should not offend anyone).

We all know Hitler used chlorine gas to murder millions of people. So, there's not a one of us who does not know how wrong this is, and should not be done to anyone. But guess what? Almost every one of you are doing the same thing to yourself, and doing it daily in most cases. You got that hot chlorinated water steaming up the shower enclosure and that chlorinated steam goes right into your lungs and into your blood stream as fast as possible.

Remember when I pointed out that YOU are the one who made YOU sick? Who told you chlorine gas was safe! Oh yeah. I forgot to mention that HUGE fact that the result of ingesting chlorine damages every cell it comes in contact with. Search the INTERNET to find information about all the various specific damage chlorine is known to do to your body. Check Wikipedia too.

Where do I buy probiotics, a carbon or fluoride water filter and a shower filter? I confess to buying them all off Ebay. Ha ha! You can also get some probiotics from Puritans Pride. – www.puritans.com And of course, there are lots of places on the INTERNET. We have bought from Puritan's Pride for almost 30 years. We were buying from Nutrition Headquarters who were later bought by Puritan's Pride. We buy vitamins, herbs, soap and other items from Puritans Pride too. We place an order every 2 or 3 months.

The shower filter we use is made by Crystal Quest. Search Ebay for KDF shower filter. Shower filters use a special carbon filter known as a KDF filter. This type shower filter uses a carbon filter which is designed for filtering hot water. If you run hot water through any carbon filter that is not specified as a KDF filter, the hot water will cause your carbon filter to dissolve. So make sure you purchase a KDF filter and don't be running hot water through any of the carbon or fluoride filters you use for your drinking and cooking water; which is connected to your kitchen faucet.

Beware that when we bought our first shower filter in early 2007, we couldn't find one at any store in this hub of commerce City of 55,000 people. Hard to believe, but it's true. And of course, SEARCH the INTERNET for the store of your choice if you don't care for Ebay.

As for a water filter for cooking and drinking water, I always recommend a disposable counter-top fluoride filter from Pure Water Essentials. This one: http://purewateressentials.com/ct00130.html It costs $100 plus shipping of around ten dollars. It lasts for years. Pure Water Essentials sells all types of water filters. So you can browse their site and find what's best for you. I have recommended this filter to everyone so far.

What about bottled water? The simple answer is... don't be a fool! Buying bottled water is foolish and a waste of money, unless there are some odd circumstances I haven't thought of. If the gas company has fracked your water supply you could need bottled water. Fracked water will ruin your water filter in no time! Bottled water contains more than water. I looked and looked and looked for bottled WATER, but could only find bottled water with several other ingredients!

The best bottled water I found was Ozarka. It has the fewest ingredients. You can get about ONE THOUSAND times as much filtered water by buying a counter top water filter than you get buying bottled water. Some bottled water is just tap water in a bottle too. And your fluoride filtered water is pure. Bottled water never is. So your body has to filter out those added ingredients. I bought bottled water one time, and that was enough to convince me to never buy any more.

Remember, the information in this book is not only to prevent and cure disease, it can and will save you lots and lots of money.

And that's the bottom line 'cause...whoops, don't want Stone Cold Steve Austin claiming I was using his catch phrase. So that's the bottom line 'cause... if I told you otherwise, I'd be lying.

6 -Poisons in Your Drinks

Now here's the subject that almost killed me and still shocks me and pisses me off sometimes…the poisons in our drinks. I have been an organic gardener since 1981, so I have eaten very healthy food all these years. I even trimmed the fat off all the meat I ate, to be safe. Sure I ate some bad foods. But it wasn't very often or very much. And even though I was the healthiest eater among family, friends and acquaintances, quite often people would say "Watch what you eat". "Oh I do" I would tell them, and it was the truth. I only had one cold/flu since 1981 and no serious illness for nearly two decades, so my health confirmed I was eating right. And guess what? I really was!

But you know what no one EVER told me? What I never told myself either? No one ever said "Watch what you DRINK". Oh how I wish with all my mind and body that someone would've told me that! Oh how I wish I had told myself that! But no one did, and I never did. I didn't tell anyone to watch what they drink either. But I was good at telling people "watch what you eat".

I know most of you are wondering what the blues blazes am I talking about! Don't feel bad about it. I felt like Columbus setting sail to sail off the edge of the earth and like Lewis and Clark westward explorations. I was heading into unknown territory! Why the very idea of thinking something bad about beloved companies who make Coke, Pepsi, Dr. Pepper, Ocean Spray, Gatorade, Welch's and the rest. All their products are verified "safe" by the FDA. But what their products had done to my health compelled and convinced me to at least consider bad things about those products.

At first I was lost as to figure out what blew out my kidneys. I tell the whole story in Chapter 8 about how I came to learn almost all the cures I have proven and learned about and what happened that forced me to face up to reality as it really is about everything I was eating, drinking or coming into contact with. I am writing this chapter to tell this part of my story in better detail than will be in Chapter 8.

When I began to learn the magnitude of how poisoned our drinks supply is, my incurable chronic kidney disease began to improve; instead of getting progressively worse and end in death. The only options doctors gave me was dialysis within 2 years and death likely shortly thereafter. I would need a kidney transplant at that point to avoid death. So I was determined to find out what caused my kidneys to fail, even though the doctors could never tell me. It was hypertension that blew my kidneys, but they couldn't tell me what caused my high blood pressure either. One doctor said it was probably salt. But none of my metabolic tests ever backed that up or even hinted to such a thing. So all I could do is wonder what caused this. I was lost as anyone could be and felt so helpless. But one day that all began to change.

As I began to pay attention to how I felt; examining, scrutinizing and analyzing how I felt all day long, I began to recognize a reoccurring bad sick feeling. I had been scrambling to find something to drink to replace the sugar soaked sweet tea I loved to guzzle down at every meal. So I got me some fruit juices. I got the ones that said they were made from concentrate. Gee. I'm about to drink some totally healthy fruit juice and not only that, it's concentrated fruit juice! Yippee. Roll out the success mat. I've got something healthy to drink, and lots of it. But then, here comes that mean a-hole, Mr. Reality and Mr. Facts to boot…and there goes my fruit juices!

The problem is that I thought concentrate meant they boiled the fruit juice down to make a concentrated form of that juice. I was wrong. The FDA guidelines for claiming something as concentrate basically means…packed with as much sugar or high fructose corn syrup as they choose to put in their products. I kept reading fruit juice cans and jars looking for any juice that was not made from concentrate. As I read the labels I keep noticing high fructose corn syrup in the ingredients. My wife and I kept throwing our hands up in disbelief about this. The reality is that **once you start trying to eliminate high fructose corn syrup, the grocery store becomes a much smaller place.**

When I started looking for fruit juices without high fructose corn syrup, I was still chugging' down the cranberry juice. I was just blind to the facts. I had been drinking this most popular brand of cranberry juice and bragged about how healthy it was for me. Of course, I hadn't read the label either. Turns out it has more sugar declared on the label than your most popular brands of soda pops. I thought, no this can't be true. Something as good for you as cranberry juice and they packed it with poison. It made no sense. It couldn't be true. OR maybe I was just full of you know what. It rhymes with mit.

So I drank some cranberry juice and within 10 minutes I had that tense sick feeling again. I realized that I had that feeling every time I drank some cranberry juice after my kidneys failed. But it was so out of place and downright insane that something so good for you was really extremely bad for you. I had been drinking a quart a day almost every day for almost 3 years. All that time I thought I was so smart to be drinking cranberry juice almost every day. I never even stopped to think it might be bad for you. I tossed out the last of the cranberry juice and kept on looking for anything without high fructose corn syrup.

Boy, what a bummer! I was down to water and milk. And at that time, I hadn't gotten my fluoride water filter I talked about in the previous chapter. At that point I was starting to make it a habit to read every label. So **I was wondering what poisons I was gonna find in my milk** and leave me with nothing but water to drink. I tried switching to 2% milk. But it tasted weak to me. While I went back and forth between whole milk and 2% milk, I researched the information about the various types of milk.

Whole milk is at least 3.25% milk fat. 2% milk is 2% milk fat. And skim and non-fat milk contain no more than 0.5% milk fat by weight. The significance of the fat content is that the growth hormones, antibiotics and other chemicals are concentrated and stored in fat cells in mammals; which includes cattle and humans. So the more fat in the milk, the more of these drugs and chemicals you will be consuming. When you try and switch from whole milk to a lower fat milk, you will probably have a hard time and want to give up. Hey, I hope you switch overnight! But most can't do that.

What I found out is that your body and mind are addicted to the chemicals you taste in whole milk. You think you like that momentary pleasure. So you have to deal with what's going on in your mind. This is true about any and every food you are addicted to. IF you crave it or make excuses for not switching to a healthier version of a product, then you are addicted to that product. I hear that about milk only second to soda pops.

Attitude and proper mind set – I want you to know that as I write this book, I have to keep trying to get the point across to you that we all naively believe our food, drinks and water supplies are really safe. I have to work hard to get it across to you that this is absolutely false. In reality, rare few food products we ingest are safe. The FDA declares products safe as long as they don't kill you quickly. So stop agreeing to do what kills you a little bit later than if you had taken cyanide pills.

It took about 5 years of regular use of a quart of cranberry juice, 20 oz. Gatorade, 3 sodas and a quart of sweet tea a day to cause my kidney failure. And I never saw it coming. Why would I? I was eating extremely healthy and drinking Gatorade to get my electrolytes and cranberry juice full of anti-oxidants and cancer preventing Lipton sweet tea.

Don't be scared. Be informed! If I skipped all these parts about attitude and mind set, you will most likely miss the boat on actually curing yourself or preventing the diseases you will get by trusting the food companies and medical professionals. You need to have a chip on your shoulder at the grocery store that pushes you to read labels in the store and never bring the poisons home in the first place. **Everything you buy is poisoned. All you CAN do is limit the amount of poisons you purchase and ingest.** And when you ingest poisons in liquid form your body digests and absorbs a far greater amount of these poisons.

What about soda pops? Sorry, it's all bad news when it comes to soda pops. The acidity of all sodas is roughly 3.0. Problem is, that your body's pH needs to be between 6.0 and 7.3. The further below 7.3 you get, the more your pH adversely affects and impedes body metabolisms. In simple words, drinking sodas makes your body ripe for disease just because of the extreme acidity. The HMF in high fructose corn syrup, hydroxymethylfurfural, has been linked to DNA damage in humans. HMF content rises as high fructose corn syrup gets warm and rises dramatically once it reaches 120° Fahrenheit.

Then add to that the sodium benzoate that has been proven to have the ability to switch off vital parts of DNA in a cell's mitochondria. And when you add vitamin C in with the sodium benzoate it causes benzene, a known carcinogenic substance. The mitochondria is called the power station of the DNA. So this damage is severe and leads to serious cell malfunction. This damage is linked to such diseases as Parkinson's disease, many neuro-degenerative diseases and most of all the whole aging process.

Now what I am about to add about sodas is my opinion from my experiences with sodas, what I have researched and what I concluded on my own. I don't have any proof beyond my opinion and experiences. So you can choose whether to believe the following. I concluded that high fructose corn syrup mutates your genes. Some have stated that high fructose corn syrup is made with genetically altered corn in a 3 step process using genetically altered enzymes. The manufacturers of this poison won't tell you exactly how it's made and advertise what seems to be a white lie recipe for high fructose corn syrup. It shouldn't surprise anyone.

They have never admitted the scientific facts about the poisons in their HFCS. They have even started calling HFCS "corn sugar" to try and hide HFCS as an ingredient in products. But it may very well be the DNA altering actions of the ingredients in sodas that I have concluded to be gene-mutating actions. I will continue being open to the facts in order to reach a final decision about this.

What is bad about sodas? DNA altering HMF, DNA altering sodium benzoate, a 3.0 acidity and possible gene-mutating high fructose corn syrup; which is also where the HMF comes from. And you get that wonderful sugar burn with every drink, and the acid also eats away at your teeth and gums. It sure didn't take any more for me to stop drinking sodas. I went from drinking at least one thousands sodas a year to somewhere around 10 to 12 sodas a year. As I look back at this, I have no doubt as to why my kidneys failed.

All these serious poisons, not to mention the fact that one 12 ounce soda pop shuts down your immune system for about 6 hours. Technically it does not shut your immune system down. It's just that your immune system is pre-occupied with trying to remove all the ingredients your body can't use. That is all it can do for about six hours. Drink a soda every 6 hours and you in essence have no immune system working to heal you. How do you have a chance against sickness in this condition!

So what about tea? Tea is really good for you. I still drink tea and have all along. We switched to Lipton decaffeinated tea, but still couldn't stand swigging down all that sugar to sweeten tea. We used less and less sugar to see if that would work. You're suppose to use 4 cups per gallon. But we only used half that amount for years. So we started using less and less. It was OK in moderation, but I wasn't liking it very well after all those years of thick sugary tea. One day we heard about an herbal sweetener called Stevia. Stevia is 30 times as sweet as sugar. We used less than a teaspoon in a gallon of tea. At first I kept saying "This tea just isn't sweet at all" and started to abandon Stevia altogether. I decided that before I did that I would do a little test. I made a gallon pitcher of tea. Poured a few ounces into a glass, unsweetened. Then I added the Stevia to the pitcher of tea. Drank one, then the other. Ah hah!

Now I could tell the Stevia really was making the tea sweet. The problem was that the tea wasn't giving my mouth that sugar burn that gives you cotton mouth, dry mouth. I then realized that I had been addicted to that sugar burn, and had been swigging down tea to get that sugar burn sensation. It's the same kind of mind addiction that all those chemicals in whole milk give you. As long as you remember that sugar burn is the proof of how bad sugar is, you will make the switch to Stevia. I'll cover this some more in the Chapter – Poisons in Your Foods, when I discuss sweeteners.

Solutions and Chapter Summary – I'm sorry to sink the Titanic about all your favorite drinks like sodas and fruit juices. But really, basically all the drink products on the market are flavored sugar waters. And most of them are packed with the worst poison of all in my experiences, research and opinion… high fructose corn syrup. You need to assume every drink product is packed with high fructose corn syrup, and check the labels to see IF you can find something that does not have HFCS.

When it comes to juices, look for products that say "NOT FROM CONCENTRATE". These words will be in plain sight. But even when the product says "NOT FROM CONCENTRATE", you still need to read the labels and see what the ingredients are. If it has high fructose corn syrup, don't buy it. The only juices we buy are Simply Orange, Florida Nature and Tropicana orange juices and Musselman's apple juice. The Tropicana orange juice in our refrigerator right now says "NEVER FROM CONCENTRATE" on the front of the cartoon. Always read the ingredients to make sure it doesn't have HFCS in it.

That's my entire findings for juices that are worth buying, if you care anything about your health. I told you already how tiny the grocery store gets once you start reading labels to eliminate high fructose corn syrup from your diet! This is one of the main reasons I wrote this book. You can try hundreds of different juices, read hundreds of juice labels…and only about 2% of the juice products available are healthy and actually safe to drink.

In addition to Simply Orange, Florida Nature and Tropicana orange juices… and Musselman's apple juice, you can drink 2% or skim milk, Unsweetened or

Stevia sweetened tea and filtered water. One juice I failed to mention was tomato juice. Tomato juice is pretty good for you. The only drawback is if you absolutely have to avoid salt, you shouldn't drink tomato juice. Tomato juice is packed heavily with salt. Tomato juice contains about 650mg of sodium per 8 ounce serving; which translates to roughly 5000mg of salt per 48 ounce can.

If you're going to drink milk, then simply drink 2% milk. If you can find it and afford it, buy Organic 2% milk. I think even Organic Whole milk would have less poisons in it than non-organic 2% milk. I drink Organic 2% milk when they have it at Kroger's. That stuff Wal-Mart sells has a slightly funky taste. That makes it suspicious to me. So I buy Organic milk only from Kroger. It's $2 a gallon more than regular milk, but well worth it. Use less milk so you buy less often. Organic milk keeps fresh weeks after regular milks have soured too.

I just recently tried that new soda pop called Sierra Mist Natural. It's a lemon lime soda that, believe it or not, does not contain high fructose corn syrup or man-made artificial sweeteners. It just contains sugar. The ingredients are carbonated water, sugar, citric acid, natural flavor and potassium citrate. Citric acid is organic. Potassium citrate is a potassium salt of citric acid. Sugar is a processed food substance and carbonated water is water that has had carbon dioxide gas under pressure dissolved in it.

So that's a pretty good soda, except for the acidic carbonated water and the empty calories of the sugar. But it doesn't have a yucky chemical taste to it compared to sodas with high fructose corn syrup and sodium benzoate. That's a tremendous improvement over all other sodas. So I'll be drinking a few of them. I'll be splitting them with my wife since that's all I drink now; just half a can at a time.

Sometimes Coke and Dr. Pepper put out a limited supply of their products that substitute pure cane sugar for high fructose corn syrup. I haven't ever been able to get any. But, it's your chance to have a soda pop without that sick high fructose corn syrup or pukey aspartame or some other man made artificial chemical sweetener.

7 -Poisons in Your Food

What do I mean by poisons in your food? I mean the chemicals that are added to food products. The most well-known are preservatives, dyes and additives of all sorts. I'm also talking about white flour, white granulated sugar, high fructose corn syrup, vegetable oils and red meat. I sometimes refer to these as poison foods. There are so many chemicals in our food supply. Quite a few of them are not necessary and are put in food products to addict you to those products. Yes, you heard me correctly. Food companies intentionally put chemicals in your food to addict you to their products. Of course, food companies won't admit this or even talk about it. But they also never talk about any proof that their chemicals are safe.

Why act like it's some secret that food companies want you to buy as much of their products as they can get you to. I've never seen any indication that they have any morals or care about you and your health one bit. All they care about is greater sales and profits to please their stockholders and their lust for money, greed. All they have to do is get FDA approval for their poisons and poison saturated products and it's all legal, approved and FDA certified safe.

As long as you don't get sick or drop dead immediately after eating their products, the FDA claims it's "safe". You are not a person or human being to corporations. You are a consumer who has what they want…your money. Has one corporation been there at the bedside of any of the millions of people their products have killed? I think NOT!

The best advice I can give anyone to inspire them to get serious about avoiding the saturation of poisons in your food is this – **Always have a chip on your shoulder when you're at the grocery store.** And no I don't mean be an a-hole to people or tackle those who look at you wrong! LOL I mean **read food labels and refuse to buy the hordes of harmful poisonous products.** I can promise you that you will begin to get furious once you start reading the labels on products after you learn about the poisons in those products.

You also need to learn what those labels mean and not be fooled by the massive trickery food companies use to trick you into buying their products. It takes more time at the grocery store, but your life is on the line and so is your health. Start right now and read all the labels on the products you already have in your home. This is exactly what my wife and I did when I blew out my kidneys in 2006.

I thought I knew the difference between healthy and harmful foods… until I started reading ALL the labels. And that was a major factor in saving my life. I'll tell you more about this later on. But for now, let's continue about food labels, what they really mean and some of the things to look for as you work to keep these poisons out of your homes and out of your bodies.

Reading labels and knowing what they mean is about the most important thing to do for finding the poisons in your food and drinks so you can avoid them.

Here's what the FDA says about the ingredient labels on products:

All the ingredients, listed in order of predominance by weight. In other words, the ingredient that weighs the most is listed first, and the ingredient that weighs the least is last.

So the first ingredient could be as much as 99% of the product. And the second ingredient could be as much as 49% of the product by weight. These are the extremes possible in any product. If a product lists any of the toxic poisons mentioned in this book in the first three ingredients, that product should be on your hit list…a product to eliminate or greatly limit and restrict its use. If the poison is toward the middle of the label, consider it a moderate health risk. If the poison is listed toward the end, consider it a mild risk if used regularly. **Reading labels MUST become a way of life.**

Even after years of reading labels we still make mistakes and buy products in every category; high risk, moderate and mild. IF I had it my way, food companies would be required to put labels on poison soaked products that say "Regular use of this product will cause diseases and eventually kill you." But hey, that would be honest. So that's NOT going to happen. Take high fructose corn syrup for example:

This DNA altering poison is in everything, and I mean everything. The most harmful products that contain high fructose corn syrup are fruit juices and soda pops. And yes, I said fruit juices. I don't know more harmful products than fruit juices and soda pops. They are not only saturated with poisons, as a liquid they are far more easily digested than any solid foods and therefore far more harmful. I went into some of the specific details about these drinks in the "Poisons in Your Drinks" chapter.

Now I will tackle some real problems with popular food items and tell you why you should avoid them and what you can do about substituting healthier products for those poisonous food products. Let's get started!

What about bread? Whole wheat or white? Well, the easy way is just to say eat whole wheat breads and flour. But most people don't know why they should choose whole wheat, and a lot of us can't even buy whole wheat buns, cakes, cookies, etc. You certainly can't find a restaurant that serves whole wheat bread, buns or rolls. Yes it's insane. But that's the reality we are forced to deal with. I have never understood why whole wheat bread is sometimes hard to find and nearly impossible to get in restaurants.

You need to tell every restaurant you do business with that you want whole wheat bread, buns, cakes and cookies, and that you will take your business elsewhere if they don't start providing it. I doubt it will do much good, even though it's the right thing to do. Restaurants are food companies too. So they had rather sell you white bread and vegetable oil soaked food than to take the time to care about the health and welfare of its customers. I don't believe restaurants care what customers want. At least I don't have any proof that they do. If you can find a restaurant that serves whole wheat bread or fries their foods in canola oil, then you've found a restaurant that at least cares a little about your health.

Now, what to buy at the grocery stores – If you're at the grocery store and see loaves of bread that claim they're whole wheat, look again. Look at the label. Most of what is called whole wheat is not. Food companies label it whole wheat, but when you read the label you see the first ingredient is "enriched wheat flour". Sounds good, right? WRONG!

What enriched wheat flour really is, is white flour with vitamins. What you have to look for is breads that list the first ingredient as "whole wheat flour" or "stone ground whole wheat flour". Otherwise it's only gonna be white flour in that bread. Tricky, misleading labeling is just one of the ways food corporations retain the level of poisons in food products while tricking you into believing their products are not only safe, but healthy and good for you. Nonsense!

Did you know that white flour is a drug? There is no such thing as a white flour plant. So where does white flour come from? It comes from wheat. Food companies take wheat and remove everything from the wheat that has real nutritional value and you get white flour. They remove the wheat bran and the wheat germ and end up with that drug called white flour. You can buy white flour real cheap. Wheat bran and wheat germ are expensive and usually have to be bought from so-called health food stores; even though you can sometimes buy wheat bran and wheat germ at your grocery store.

It's shocking to learn how food companies strip wheat of all its nutritional value and sell what's left, white flour. White flour eventually causes diarrhea and intestinal bleeding. This is caused by lack of fiber, and of course, if you've ever taken a slice of white bread and smashed it into as small a ball as you can, then you have already seen the proof of how white flour has no fiber. You eat the white bread and then scramble to get more fiber in your diet; when all you have to do is eat whole wheat bread and make sure it's really whole wheat. Then you would have plenty of fiber.

Trying to avoid white flour can become a real pain in the ass because of how limited the supply of real whole wheat bread is, and because of how food companies tend to rely on that drug called white flour to addict you to their products. You buy a greasy burger at a fast food restaurant and it comes on white bread so it doesn't interfere with the taste of the grease soaked burger. Whole wheat has some nutritional value, so it also has some taste to it. You want a whole wheat cake, but can never find a whole wheat cake mix. You want whole wheat cookies, but nobody sells them. You want whole wheat buns, but you can hardly ever find them either. So what's a person to do?

You can always get a bread maker for about $70-100 and make your own. Or you can substitute whole wheat flour for white flour in recipes. You can also add some whole grains like crushed flax seed or whole wheat flour to the recipe. Adding wheat bran and wheat germ to recipes also brings some nutritional value to recipes. One thing we do is use half whole wheat flour in raisin bread. You're suppose to use bread flour. But you can use whole wheat flour as long as you add a teaspoon of wheat gluten for each cup of whole grain flour.

So when it comes to buying bread, remember to read the labels and only buy bread whose first ingredient is whole wheat flour or Stone ground whole wheat; and not to be fooled by the hordes of breads that say whole wheat on the package, but the first ingredient is white flour with vitamins; known as enriched wheat flour. There are also other whole grain breads besides wheat, like rye and multi-grain breads. When I eat out, it's at Subway's 9 times out of 10. And I always get multi-grain bread for every sandwich; not to mention the pile of chopped fresh veggies on every sandwich.

If I haven't made it clear, do not eat white bread. That means no white bread, hot dog buns, hamburger buns, dinner rolls, crescent rolls, cakes, cobblers, dough nuts, pastries and on and on and on. Look for whole wheat versions of all of these food items or do without them, or at least eat them in moderation and don't make a habit of doing so. It's not worth the damage to your health; especially when you could be eating wholesome whole grain products with the fiber and nutrients your body needs. You'll feel a lot better about yourself and enjoy a much healthier body the more you choose healthy foods, and the less you choose the unhealthy foods that the grocery store shelves are packed with.

Sure you gotta spend time to learn and do all of this! But isn't your life worth the effort? Is your health worth the effort? Isn't your financial health worth it? And aren't the lives of your family and loved ones and their health and well-being worth the effort? Making these changes in diet and lifestyle certainly is hard at first, mainly because you are so set in your ways. It's up to you to do the right thing for you and your families. I know you can do this. And the more you learn and put into practice, the more positive results you get, the more you want to learn and get to doing. And you WILL get those results as long as you make the effort.

Meat, meat and more meat – What meat should I eat? The best answer is none, you shouldn't eat meat at all. I'll go into detail about red meat in just a few minutes. But for now, let's learn something about meat in general. Meat is dead animal flesh. We fatten animals on corporate farms, feeding and injecting these animal with all kinds of drugs and chemicals, kill them systematically, skin them and cut their dead flesh into pieces and parts; which is what you buy at the grocery store. We make up all kinds of names for these dead animal parts and flesh to try and fool ourselves into thinking we are eating something good and healthy. Millions of Americans even take dead animal parts and smoke them on their charcoal grills; saturating them with smoke and soot that tastes good, but is poison to your body. We eat the dead flesh of cows, pigs, turkeys and chickens. Quite a few people eat deer, elk, bison and an array of other dead animal flesh and parts.

Don't get me wrong. IF you can get any meat that comes from outside the corporate food companies, that meat has avoided the saturation of chemicals that are in all meat sold by corporations. You can't chase a deer down and make him drink soda pops or fruit juice to poison the deer meat. You can't inject wild deer with antibiotics and growth hormones either. The only chance of wild animals having poisons in their systems is if they have been drinking or eating chemicals that come from the massive pollution of our air, water and land by corporations.

But humans are not supposed to be meat eaters. We don't have the teeth to be meat eaters. Meat eaters have some spiked teeth so they can rip and shred meat. Humans do not. Human teeth are for chewing vegetation and fish. But no one ever talks about this, no matter how many so-called health books you read. No…we just can't bear to be honest about things. The truth might offend someone, or cut back on the sales of their book or other things. I wouldn't even begin writing this book for a few years because of that fact.

I have been attacked, slandered, hated, threatened and even had a guy pull a gun on me in Public for stating some of these facts. I have been warned by dozens of people that I am going to get someone killed by telling them how to cure themselves of diseases. All of this is insane and complete nonsense on their part. How flax seed oil, fish oil or vitamins could kill someone is unfounded and unheard of! But quite honestly, a lot of these lunatics are in the medical profession and/or their christianity has taught them to ignore GOD's natural cures in favor of the sorcery and quackery the medical profession invented the past 75 years. Even if there is no GOD, man has been using cures from nature since man first existed. So telling anyone anything besides "go to the doctor" is what they pretend is me trying to get people killed.

Problem with that nonsense is that I have never told anyone NOT to go to the doctor. I only tell people that IF they want to be cured, going to the doctor is not the thing to do, since doctors have no cures. If you lose your car keys, do you look on the TV and not find them and give up and never drive your car again! NO YOU DON'T. You keep looking until you find them! And people want to accuse ME of trying to get people killed for telling you to do the same thing when it comes to your health and life! Keep going to your sorcerers disguised as doctors WHILE you cure yourself. Having a doctor to send blood tests to the lab will help you realize that you really are curing yourself, preventing disease or at the least, getting better. But I'll have a lot more to say about all this in Chapter 8. Let's get back to Poisons in our Food.

The American diet – Dead cow flesh – Everyone is on that savages' diet called the American diet; which is red meat. This country gobbles down one meal after another of that red meat that is soaked with growth hormones, antibiotics, other drugs, chemicals from the food cows eat and parasites. Red meat increases the risk of cancer, heart disease, Alzheimer's, stomach ulcers and an array of other conditions. But this country just keeps right on scarfing down the red meat. And it's the main food for almost the entire country.

The fat from red meat ends up clogging your veins and arteries. This fat along with vegetable oil is the major factor in creating clogged arteries and veins and raising blood pressure by accumulating on the walls of your veins and arteries. Once this plaque breaks off it can easily lodge in your brain or heart and cause a stroke or heart attack.

I got to tell you, it just bobbles the mind how we all stuff this garbage down our own throats and no matter how many consequences we suffer for doing so, we go right on doing it day after day to no end. Why? Because we refuse to face reality as it is. So we never even think corporations would be allowed to poison everyone for any reason, including the main reason most of these poisons are in your food, drinks and water - increasing corporate profits. Your life and health are irrelevant. We are not even human beings to the corporations. We are consumers, consumers of their products. And the only thing that means to corporations is that you are the ones they work to addict to their products. And as long as you buy their products there is nothing they COULD do that would be wrong. NO WAY!

Their poisons AND the products they use as the delivery device for those addicting poisons are FDA Certified safe. LOL All I can do is laugh at the extreme corruption of the FDA and the corporations. You need to re-evaluate your opinion of corporations who poison you in order to create changes in the human mind that cause your food addictions. As a matter of fact, all the food corporations are really doing is laughing all the way to the bank, while the medical industry laughs all the way to the bank too and thanks the food corporations for creating 75% of their business. They rake in the billions of dollars from you, while you suffer, lose your lives and end up bankrupt because of this transfer of wealth from you to the billion dollar corporations! And red meat is a major factor in all of this.

If dead cow flesh is so good for you as those who sell red meat claim, then why do you call dead cow flesh beef, steak, hamburger meat, hot dogs and all those other names substituted for dead cow flesh? It doesn't LOOK like they're trying to mislead, they ARE misleading you. Maybe if you would call something what it actually is, you might not be so quick to eat so much of it or not at all. And that's what's best for you. If you're going to eat dead cow flesh, I suggest you stick to Ground Chuck. Ground Chuck is ground beef without nearly as much fat. It's that fat, greasy taste you get addicted to eating red meat.

Now, I could go on about how bad red meat really is, but I've given you the information you need to make a rational decision to cut out red meat. If you can't cut out red meat now that you have faced the facts, then you are addicted to red meat. So to get off the red meat, you would have to pay attention to what's going on in your head while you are eating red meat. That's where the addiction is. And that's where you have to fight all these food addictions, in your head and way of thinking.

Your body goes to work fighting all those chemicals and fat in red meat as soon as it gets into your body. And, your body can't rid itself of those chemicals completely under normal circumstances. So do yourself and your own health a big favor... stop eating red meat! But since I know how hard it is to stop cold turkey, I recommend working to limit your red meat intake until you no longer eat red meat at all. I have already done this. But I do eat a pound or two of Ground Chuck in a pot of soup or a home cooked hamburger. I haven't eaten at McDonald's but once in the past 25 years, and that was when my wife and I were in Memphis for a major event. I have had my cholesterol checked and it is well within normal and I have no problems associated with cholesterol or fat. I hope you get off the red meat AND the vegetable oils that are clogging your veins and arteries and disabling and killing tens of thousands of people every year in this country.

One other tip that can help is about outdoor charcoal grilling! I use to grill outdoors every few weeks until my kidneys blew out. But that all came to a screeching halt after that happened. I love eating charcoal grilled chicken, hamburgers, steaks, hot dogs and vegetable shishkabobs. But it's easy to see why it's all bad for you. First of all, it's bad enough that you're eating dead cow flesh. But on top of the meat already being drug saturated, you smoke it with burning charcoal! Gee, why not just stuff a wash cloth down your throat! Only difference would be the delay in taking your breath away and the time of death! Maybe you can just use the rule of doing these things in moderation and stop being so gung ho about stuffing as much red meat and charcoal grilled meat down your throat?

Even the chicken, turkey and fish become repulsive to your body once they're heavily smoked on the outdoor grill. So think about what you are really doing and stop lying to yourself about red meat being safe and smoking that meat being safe. Red meat is bad for you, and smoking it compounds that negative impact on your health. This country is obsessed with eating things that are very bad for you, while talking about the great food they are eating! This book seeks to cure you of that delusion and get you back on the road to healthy living and add days, weeks, months and years to your life and the lives of your family and other loved ones.

Vegetable oils – Canola Oil – Olive Oil or what? The simple answer to that question is olive oil. Olive oil is the best oil to use. But since it's quite costly it's not a practical solution for most people. Vegetable oils are always the cheapest. So people tend to lean heavily toward vegetable oils to cook with. But is your health and life really worth the savings in money? No it is not!

If you're old enough, you can remember how no one really said a thing about vegetable oils being bad for you until the past 20 years or less. But can you remember when no one thought cigarettes were bad for you either? Yea. **Doctors would go on TV and tell you not only that cigarettes were safe for you, but that cigarettes had quite a few health benefits.** Sounds crazy right? Totally crazy, right? It wasn't back then when they were doing this. There was no Public outcry against cigarettes at that time. People trusted their sorcerers with their new name "doctor", but not as much as people do now. They were pretty rational at that time, but were still tricked by the tobacco industry and the medical profession about cigarettes. And it's been the same story about vegetable oil and high fructose corn syrup.

You all choke down gobs and gobs of vegetable oils. It's bad enough that you cook in vegetable oil, but most of the vegetable oil you consume doesn't come from the foods soaked in vegetable oil that you fry at home. The biggest source of vegetable oils is in processed foods like Oreo cookies, Twinkies, Potato chips, breads, cakes, pies, peanut butter and margarine! I'm not picking on just these food products. The grocery store shelves are packed with vegetable oil saturated food products just like the ones I just named.

You need to look for trans-fat content on the label and avoid any products that have ANY trans-fats at all. In the ingredients, look for partially hydrogenated oils. Trans-fats are a byproduct which is created during partial dehydrogenation. But beware! Just because the label lists trans-fats as zero, they can still have trans-fats. Food manufacturers only list trans-fats above zero if the product contains at least 0.5 grams of trans-fats per serving.

They even fix the labeling per serving many times so they can claim their products contain zero trans-fats on the label. Trans-fats reduce the amount of good, HDL, cholesterol in your body. So if the ingredients list partially dehydrogenated oil of any kind, avoid that product. Do not buy it. But no matter how well you solve this problem in your own household, you still scarf down good amounts of vegetable oils when you eat any restaurant food.

There is no need to single out any one restaurant or many restaurants! Your whole problem with eating restaurant food is that none of it is healthy. They'll put out a salad bar at some places instead of cooking in canola oil, using whole wheat flour, honey and no high fructose corn syrup. They are in business to make money and make as much money as they can within the Laws of this country. The problem there is how we don't have a real government in this country any more. So it doesn't matter how bad these substances in the food supply are, as long as it's FDA approved, there is no government to do a thing about it. Everything you eat in restaurants are cooked in vegetable oils. The damage those oils do to your body creates that craving for all the poison soaked foods and drinks you consume. It's that added taste that vegetable oils give foods that are cooked in vegetable oils.

You think that chicken is good for you from that famous fried chicken restaurant, even though it's soaked in those artery clogging vegetable oils. Hey, I love their chicken. But I haven't eaten it but twice in the past four years. About the only thing you can do about this is stop eating restaurant food; especially the big chain franchise restaurants. At smaller local restaurants you should tell the managers and owners of their restaurants that you want your food cooked in canola oil and want a better choice of drinks with no high fructose corn syrup. Let them know it's a serious health need for you and your family. But don't let anyone distract you from your choices to avoid consuming foods and drinks that are bad for your health.

The only restaurant whose food I eat is almost always SubWay. I always get my sandwiches on multi-grain bread. I usually get the Orchard Chicken. It's like a chicken salad, but has cranberries, apple and black olives on it. Of course, you can get whatever you want on your sandwich, but cranberries are only on the Orchard Chicken that I know of. I also get the Oven Roasted Chicken as my second favorite, but sometimes will get a Philly Steak and Cheese or a Meatball sandwich. Although these sandwiches aren't as healthy as the Orchard Chicken, they come topped with lots of fresh sliced veggies.

And having the multi-grain bread makes SubWay the healthiest restaurant eating I know of. I might break down once every month or two and get a Veggie Lovers pizza from Pizza Hut, but Subway is easily our favorite restaurant. I like to eat some egg rolls from the Chinese restaurants too from time to time.

But hey…eating out costs at least twice as much for the same food if you cook it at home. And with the very little chance of eating anything healthy from 99% of the restaurants, eating at home is the all-around best idea for sure. So eating at home is always going to be more healthy and cheaper than any food you can get in restaurants; especially the well-known fast food chains.

Olive oil is the best oil to use by far. Extra virgin olive oil is the best olive oil.

Virgin olive oil is almost as good a quality as Extra Virgin Olive oil, but is not. I always buy Extra Virgin Olive oil for about $6 a quart. My wife uses olive oil to oil the skillet to cook grilled sandwiches and other light oiling cooking jobs. You can also whip up some mayonnaise using olive oil. It will last about 2 weeks in the refrigerator. Olive oil has many health benefits which I will go in to as we go along. Olive oil even has some great health care uses I bet most of you are unaware of! Always keep some olive oil in your home, and use it efficiently to make it go a long way. If money is no object, use it generously. The more you use olive oil, the greater good you've done for yourself.

The best all-around oil is canola oil. Although it doesn't have the extensive health benefits that olive oil has, canola oil is about 25% the cost of Extra Virgin Olive Oil. Canola oil costs the same as vegetable oils. With that fact in mind, I cannot for the life of me, understand why anyone would buy vegetable oil instead of canola oil! There is no known damage which canola does to your body. On the contrary! There are lots of people who take a tablespoon or two of canola oil for their hearts most days. Canola oil has the lowest saturated fat content of all oils; including olive oil. It is very high in unsaturated fats too. Because of canola oil's excellent health benefits, I suggest you read more about canola oil and olive oil, and SEARCH the INTERNET too.

Also, peanut oil has the most (good) monounsaturated fat other than olive and canola oil. Sunflower oil is also a better choice than vegetable oils, but still lags behind olive, canola and peanut oil as far as overall health benefits. But it's still a much better choice than artery clogging vegetable oils. So avoid using vegetable oils by making the healthier choice at the grocery store. Stock up when it's on sale.

Sugars and Sweeteners – Here's the information most people are interested in more than any other food information. It really does get confusing when you're trying to make healthy choices about sugar and other sweeteners. But just like all the food products we buy as consumers, healthy choices are hard to come by. Food companies are little to no help here either! The only healthy choices I know of among sweeteners is Stevia, raw honey and pure cane sugar. Since sugar is the most common sweetener of all, let's start there.

I told you to use pure cane sugar. But you have to pay precise attention to the term being used. You will often see, if not always, that white granulated sugar is called pure cane sugar. But it is NOT! Pure cane sugar is brown. Now you probably think you should buy brown sugar then, huh? Well don't! Brown sugar is a type of sugar. Brown sugar is just white granulated sugar sprayed with molasses. Brown sugar is NOT pure cane sugar as far as naming and labeling go. Confusing, right? Pure Cane sugar is named Pure Cane sugar and it is always BROWN. But Pure Cane sugar is not named or labeled as "brown sugar". **So only buy precisely named brown "Pure Cane sugar", not white.**

White granulated sugar is made by processing sugar cane. They remove everything that is good in the sugar cane and end up with white granulated sugar. During that process, they add sulfur dioxide, phosphoric acid and calcium hydroxide to the liquid cane sugar that eventually becomes granulated white sugar. White sugar is toxic to your body and weakens your body's ability to fight off disease and also overloads your lymph system. Your lymph systems and nodes are part of your body's immune system. It's also a well-known fact that white granulated sugar (sucrose) causes tooth decay, and is a major factor in obesity and diabetes.

I have always referred to white granulated sugar as a drug. Many others also call it a chemical. Your body sees it as a toxin that has to be removed. White granulated sugar, sucrose, has no real nutritional value. It only gives you empty calories. And those empty calories are high octane fuel inside your body. With all that sugar firing up inside your body as instant body fuel, energy, it should come as no surprise how that process is damaging your body inside! That resulting heartburn should come as no surprise either.

Hey...if you stick your hand over a fire it gets burned. Scarf down white granulated sugar and heartburn is almost certain; and more so the older you get! Avoiding white granulated sugar, sucrose, is a pretty humongous task in this country. The only consolation to consuming white granulated sugar is that it's not high fructose corn syrup. If you just gotta eat sweets, at least make sure it does not have high fructose corn syrup! White sugar is only the lesser of two evils.

We have not bought any white granulated sugar in over four years. We do buy the brown pure can sugar from time to time. We only started doing this in the past year though. Remember, brown pure cane sugar does still have the molasses in it and is the least processed of sugar cane sugars. So it is the healthiest of the cane sugars. If you just gotta continue with recipes that call for sugar, then substitute brown pure cane sugar for white granulated sugar in your recipes. There are a lot of restaurants that make their own ice cream using liquid pure cane sugar. You can tell it doesn't have that sugar bite you get eating white granulated sugar and high fructose corn syrup.

Brown pure cane sugar will cost you more than white granulated sugar, and it should too! Hey...you're getting sugar that has no bad health consequences, besides all those calories, and that's the most important thing when it comes to what you eat and drink. Sometimes you can find brand named Cokes, Dr. Pepper and others that use pure cane sugar instead of high fructose corn syrup. But none of them make them a regular product you can buy year round. I've bought root beer flavored sodas, like sarsaparilla, in natural food stores, and I can tell the difference real well. But like all healthy products, they're hard to find. Healthy products will be hard to find as long as the food corporations continue to be obsessed with soaking their products with whatever poisons will addict you to their products the best.

Fructose is a better choice than white granulated sugar. Although fructose rhymes with sucrose, the name for white granulated sugar, fructose is twice as sweet per serving as sucrose. Fructose is not high fructose corn syrup either. And at this time I can't really say whether fructose is bad for you. I can only say there are healthier choices than fructose. You will find fructose in Gatorade. I keep seeing another derivative name for the sugar they put in Gatorade. So I backed off drinking Gatorade except for drinking some during hot weather.

Another familiar sweetener you see on products is Sucralose. Sucralose is the sweetener family name for a brand named product called Splenda. Although Splenda, Sucralose, is the least harmful of the man-made sweeteners, I don't use it. I don't use any of the artificial sweeteners. I have researched some other sweeteners, but haven't found any that I could trust. Aspartame is some bad crap! Some sources say that Aspartame turns to formaldehyde about 80 degrees. I don't really know, even though it's very easy for me to believe that. I'm not using any product with Aspartame in it. End of story.

Honey is another product that needs some precise information when you're buying it. You can't just pick any honey if you care about your health. You should only buy raw honey. Raw honey has not been processed. It takes honey a lot longer to start turning into a thick substance. Processed honey is always clear golden brown. Raw honey is golden brown too, but is cloudy instead of clear. Those beneficial bacteria in raw honey created this cloudiness. **Again, do your research into the many health benefits of raw honey, and do your INTERNET SEARCHes.** It's hard to find raw honey in grocery stores. You should expect to pay $7 or $8 a quart when you do. I buy raw honey by the gallon for $26. It comes from a local bee farm. Use half as much raw honey as sugar if you substitute raw honey in recipes. But trying to sweeten your tea with raw honey is not really practical; although you can certainly do so if you can afford it.

When it comes to sweetening tea, we always use Stevia. Stevia is an herb that is about 30 times as sweet as sugar. Stevia has no calories too. Stevia also has no impact on diabetics, since Stevia does not affect blood sugar levels. So Stevia is an excellent healthy choice as a sweetener. When we make sweet tea at home, we use about 1/8 teaspoon per gallon of Lipton decaffeinated tea. We spend about $40 a year for enough Stevia to sweeten our tea. I drink a lot of tea, and I am thrilled to be doing so without swigging down all that white granulated sugar I drank for decades! What an improvement! If you try sweetening your tea with Stevia after having grown use to sugar sweetened tea, it won't taste very good to you at first. You won't get that sugar bite that happens to you from drinking sugar sweetened tea. So that makes you tend to think the Stevia isn't sweetening very good.

What you have to do to dispel this fallacy is this: Make your tea as you always do. Before adding the Stevia, pour 2 or 3 ounces of the unsweetened tea into a glass. Then add the Stevia to the freshly made pitcher of tea and pour some of it into a glass. Drink the unsweetened tea, then the Stevia sweetened tea. You can tell the Stevia sweetened tea IS sweetening the tea. But it's doing so without the harmful sugar bite you get from white granulated sugar, not to mention the case of "cotton mouth" you get from it! I love my Stevia sweetened tea. I did without tea after my kidneys failed, just to avoid all that sugar in liquid form. But thanks to Stevia I've been able to drink my tea AND not have any concern about the tea doing any harm to my health.

And one last thing...when I say you should drink plenty of water, that's doesn't include tea or anything that contains water. Drink all the Stevia sweetened tea you want. But don't count a bit of that tea as water.

Another sweetener you need to know about is Xylitol. Xylitol has 2/3 as many calories as white granulated sugar, but is safe for diabetics. Xylitol is found in a lot of fruits and vegetables in the fiber. Xylitol is a sugar alcohol. The most well-known use of Xylitol is for dental purposes. Xylitol kills the bacteria that cause gum disease and cavities. You will see it used in some sugarless gums too. As a matter of fact, when I get a tooth ache the first thing I do is grab a couple of Xylitol mints and slide them around the affected area and let them dissolve. It helps a great deal every time. You can get Xylitol in gum or mint form, and in toothpastes.

Eggs – There's not a lot of choices when it comes to eggs. The USDA classifies eggs as meat due to their high protein content. Just because some eggs are brown doesn't mean they are healthier than white eggs. You have to make sure those brown eggs are actually organic eggs. To comply with USDA requirements to be able to label eggs as organic, the eggs have to come from chickens that have been fed organic feed, are free of antibiotics, as well as better standards for the welfare of the chickens. The first thing you will find about the taste of organic eggs is how smooth they taste.

Organic eggs don't have that chemical bite that regular eggs do. You will begin to recognize that chemical bite in regular eggs after you've eaten organic eggs for a few weeks. It's this chemical bite or burn that I focus on while I'm eating anything, in order to recognize how poisonous or healthy any food item is. I am extremely good at this too. There have been times when my wife bought some bad food product, and I used this ability and told her it has to have high fructose corn syrup. And sure enough, it does.

It used to be hard for me to eat eggs. Even before I knew that bitter after taste was the chemicals in the eggs, I barely ate any eggs because of that. A better choice than regular eggs is Eggland Eggs. Eggland Eggs are organic eggs. These eggs come from chickens that are fed an organic vegetarian diet. For complete information on Eggland Eggs visit

http://www.egglandsbest.com/egglands-eggs/faq/our-eggs.aspx

In this book so far I have touched on the tricks food corporations use to trick you into buying their products. Some of the most popular labeling scams are using terms such as Low fat, Low salt, Low Calorie, Organic, All Natural, Diet and From Concentrate. But as you'll find out, these terms are misleading and downright false as common sense goes.

Take the Low fat, Low calorie and Low salt labeling scam. If a product contains all three of these ingredients and advertises one of these terms on the label, then the label is correct and legal. So no problem, right? No, you are wrong! If a product label says Low Salt, but has sugar and fat in it too, the food companies add about twice as much sugar and fat as the regular version of the same product! But hey, at least they didn't lie on the label. They just didn't tell you on the label that it also had twice as much sugar and fat too!

You should read the label of the regular version of any product and compare it to the Low fat, Low calorie and/or Low Salt version of that product to confirm these facts. When I first started trying to avoid salt and sugar, I read hundreds of labels of products using these labeling terms and 100% of them confirmed these facts for me. I then ceased to buy any and all products with these labeling terms and so did some friends of mine.

So unless you have some specific condition that requires you to avoid salt, sugar or fat, then stick to buying the regular versions of these products. But make sure the regular version is a healthy choice, or never put it in your grocery basket and bring it home. That's where **the front line on healthy eating and avoiding poisons is - right there in the grocery store reading those labels.**

Don't be fooled by other labeling tricks either, like Organic. I've pointed out some places you can trust the organic label term. But often times, organic doesn't mean organic. And it's left up to each one of us to sort this trickery out for ourselves. The same is true about the labeling terms Natural and All Natural. You also see the term natural ingredients as well, to convey a meaning of healthy food. But with all these terms, even the ingredients listed on the label itself will give you the proof to contradict these terms on most of these food and drink products. You begin to find out what the food companies are pretending to be natural in their tiny world.

Rare few of us would ever agree with the vast majority of the food and drinks corporations' idea of natural, All Natural and natural ingredients! **And these misleading labeling terms are fooling lots of you into continuing to**

use the same unhealthy products you always buy, by including one of these new misleading label marketing tricks/terms.

But in spite of all of this, you still have that wonderful fruit juice you love to drink. Yea, it's the one that says "Contains 100% Fruit Juice". I'm laughing now as I do just about every time I see that term on a product. If it's "100% Fruit Juice", then it contains ONLY fruit juice, right? Nope. Again…Read the label and see if the juice is the only ingredient. If not, you have your proof about this misleading labeling term. When I see that term I always think "Yea, I bet you took a little bit of "100% Fruit Juice" and put it in that product. But what's all that other crap in there!"

Don't forget the whole wheat labeling trick where they call their products whole wheat by using white flour enriched with vitamins. Only buy those that say whole wheat flour or stoned ground whole wheat flour. Buy the brown pure cane sugar, not the white granulated sugar labeled as pure cane sugar. Don't be fooled by the new term for high fructose corn syrup, which is "corn sugar". They just changed the name…even though I had such wonderful (sarcastically saying) things to say about corn sugar under its real name – high fructose corn syrup. Like this.…

It's just an adorable name. High…oh yes. I love to be high! Fructose… ahh, it's SO SO SWEET. Corn…yummy yummy corn! Syrup…so thick and sweet, like me! Ba hum bug. Gag me with that poison and blow out my kidneys and almost kill me. Not so uplifting, sweet, yummy thick a product as the name implies. HFCS should be called Heinous Freakin Causer of Sickness!

There has been lots of information about the negative effects of MSG, but food companies continue to use MSG. So you have to read the labels and do not buy products with MSG. Food manufacturers try to hide the fact that their products contain MSG by listing ingredients that contain MSG, but not the MSG itself. So avoid products if they contain free glutamate to insure your best possibility of avoiding MSG. Besides MSG, there are thousands of chemicals in food and drink products. My aim was to focus on how to reduce the total amount of poisons entering your body.

This is why I am not including a long drawn out explanation about the many other poisons in your food and drinks, or in our water supplies and personal hygiene items. I have given you a powerful guide that will result in you reducing the amount of poisons getting into your body.

Remember, it's toxins, also known as free radicals and poisons, that cause almost all disease. So eliminating poisons is the action that reduces the amount of disease your body develops. I've even heard doctors state the fact that toxins, free radicals, cause many diseases. I just haven't ever seen a doctor with the desire to trace that toxin back to its source. As sad as it actually is, your doctor can't make no money if he solves that problem; cures that disease by eliminating the poisons causing the disease or condition.

It's all up to each of you to use the power of knowledge in order to find your way through all the deceit that hurts us, but can't do a thing to change these food and drinks corporations. And that's what this book can do for you - guide you through all the things that stand in your way, to keep you eating according to corporate advertising and misleading labeling, and the most important facts you need to make the serious changes concerning all the products you buy that you consume.

I will not suggest that you try to talk with any of the food corporations or anyone in the government in pursuit of solving or diminishing this plague of poison induced sickness and disease affecting every human and animal in this country. Our humanity limits us time wise.

So use your time to read labels while you are in the grocery store. Work on recognizing the foods your mind craves when you are addicted to a food product. You have to understand that you can't wipe out all the poisons overnight! You have to start somewhere and keep learning progressively. Search the INTERNET for lots and lots of information on every subject and item. Look for information that repeats itself time after time while you're doing your searches and research. Cut back on eating out to avoid eating unhealthy. Cut down on charcoal grilling and the amount of meat you grill each time. The less poisons you put in to your body, the less health problems you will have.

I also didn't spend time going over the details of the benefits of eating fresh fruits and vegetables. To me, that's real simple. Eat all the fresh fruits and vegetables you can. Just make sure you wash them real good. I even take each grape I eat and wipe it off real good with a paper towel.

To see for yourself what good this does, eat a few grapes and focus on the taste. Then wipe off a few grapes with a paper towel and eat them. Then eat some grapes without wiping them off and notice that slight bitter taste each grape has. That's the poisons the grapes are soaked in that you are tasting.

So wash all that fruit and vegetables extra good and eat all you want. And buy organic produce to reduce those poisons as much as possible. And, Buy fresh over frozen, and frozen over canned.

8 - The Details of My "Chronic" Kidney Disease Dialysis, Death? OR Cure Myself?

Well, here we are on Chapter 8, the chapter I have referred to a few times in previous chapters. This is where I tell my story about how I came to know most of the facts and truths I have been writing in this book and sharing with people in my daily life. Now I know that most of you have been wondering about some things. Like, how did I come to know all these things I'm talking about in this book? What are my credentials? Why should you listen to me, much less believe me? Do I think I'm smarter than doctors? And...probably a few other questions like that.

You may have noticed that I didn't give you information about my education or college degrees, where I studied medicine and other things like that. The reason is because I am not a licensed doctor, have no medical degree or college degree. And I only think I'm smarter than doctors when it comes to curing disease.

Wait. I meant, I AM smarter than doctors when it comes to curing disease. I proved that first, then started admitting that. You will understand how true that is before this chapter is over. It's up to you to decide who to believe when it comes to the subject of cures for disease. You can keep listening to doctors who don't have cures for much of anything at all, OR you might consider listening to someone who has actually cured themselves or others of diseases and medical conditions; including chronic diseases. I'm not really asking you to choose. Hey, if your doctor already cured you, you don't need my help. Let me know. I honestly know of no one who has been cured by a doctor. And boy I have looked and looked and looked. You do that when your life is on the line.

I'm a pretty open minded person. So I'll try something to see if it works. I often joke that if clipping clothes pins to my nose will cure me of a disease, I'll wear clothes pins on my nose until I'm cured. Ha ha! An open mind is a requirement if you're going to prevent disease and cure yourself of disease. Now, if you have clothes pins on your nose, please, take them off!

The story leading up to this book really began in 1981 when I started taking an interest in eating a little healthier and began doing organic gardening. I learned a lot of wonderful things over the years since then. But I didn't have any proof there were any cures, except from doctors. I never got a cure for anything when I was growing up. I never heard of doctors curing anyone of anything either. But like everyone in this country, when you get sick you go to the doctor. So when I made my first doctor's appointment in October 2006 I assumed I would be cured by the doctors. I couldn't wait to get to the doctor, as bad as I felt; even though I had no need for them, except for one trip to the emergency room in 1996 for my 3rd bladder stone attack, up until that time.

I had the flu for 4 days one time from 1981 up to this very day too. So my experience with sickness was very limited to say the least. But from about 2000 until late 2006, I blindly poisoned myself with at least 3 sodas a day, sometimes adding an extra icy quart of soda pop to that total, a 20 ounce Gatorade every day, a quart of the most popular brand cranberry juice; along with my quart of tea a day at meals...sweet tea. I didn't start out drinking all that every day back in 2000. I gradually built that entire mess of bad habits for a couple of years and then sometime in 2003 I was drinking all that soda, juice, Gatorade and sweet tea. Big deal huh?

Only thing I thought about it was how brilliant I was for drinking all that cancer fighting tea, that healthy ole cranberry juice, and good ole Gatorade to get my electrolytes. I never thought for a minute that any of those drinks were hurting me in any way. Healthy organic food and healthy drinks. Ah, is this Heaven! I really thought I was doing great. But in early 2006 I started feeling like crap. My lower back would ache all the time.

I had some back problems, but always managed to work them out within a few days. So this never-ending back pain was confusing me, since it was not going away. I continued to do what I could for back pain. I tried everything I could think of to relieve the pain in my lower back. I used an inversion table, Gazelle, Lifting weights, walking, heating pad, massages and lots more. But that aching back pain continued to persist.

Now when June came that year, 2006, my throat began to bleed one afternoon. I felt something tickle my throat, and when I coughed I hacked out blood. I thought it was my gums bleeding as they use to do every day. But when I started to try and isolate where the blood was coming from, I realized it was coming from my throat. I got a bit scared when I realized that I must have throat cancer. I kept trying to clear the blood out of my mouth and throat, but it kept coming. My throat bled and bled for 16 straight hours. I laid on the bed with a large plastic blue glass and spit blood in it for that entire 16 hours. I spit out a lot of clots, coagulated blood, in that 16 hours. I fell asleep finally and when I woke up, my throat wasn't bleeding. I drank water to wash the blood taste out of my mouth and that was the end of it for the time being.

After that throat bleeding episode in June, I still had the pain in my lower back. It would get worse, then better, then worse again until the first week of October 2006. I woke up one night right after 2 A.M. to go to the bathroom. I had to piss so bad I was hurting to go. As I was pissing, I felt like I was going to pass out and as I did, I looked down and saw my pee was real pink to reddish in the toilet and all the sudden a clump comes out and drops in the toilet. I dropped to my knees instantly, fell on my face and started to pass out.

I regained my vision before I completely blacked out and started crawling out of the bathroom, through our band room, to my bed. I started mumbling to my wife, who was asleep, "Sandra, Sandra. Help me. Help me".

She woke up and freaked out at what she saw, but tried to help me. She helped me up and helped me lay down on the bed. I had no idea what was wrong with me, what caused it or what to do for myself. So I just laid in bed while my wife sat up the rest of the night to keep an eye on me in case anything else happened, worse than what had already occurred. I fell asleep a couple of hours later, and my wife dosed off once she saw me fall asleep. Neither one of us slept very long.

We got up for the day between 6 and 7 A.M. And that's when the evil fun really got going. I spent the next week standing over the toilet at first. Then I had to start sitting on the toilet to try and pee dozens of times a day, since I was getting tired of standing half the day trying to pee. I didn't really need to pee all the time. It just felt like I needed to. You know how it is…you take a leak to relieve yourself. But no matter how much I tried to relieve myself, relief never came that week. I barely slept. On my best days that week I would sleep maybe 2-3 hours. I would try to go to sleep. But I would just lay in bed, unable to fall asleep, and end up getting up and standing over the toilet waiting for some relief. But no relief.

I can't pinpoint whether it was just a week or more than a week this went on, while I waited for the day of my first doctor's appointment in about 30 years. I was dazed and shocked and in my own little world just hoping for a few seconds of relief from the constant body aches and impulses to pee dozens of times a day. My wife was in shock too. She had never seen me in that shape and was just so naive about how bad a shape I was in. And she had been with me the whole time I had my four bladder stone attacks 10 years earlier from 1993-1996.

I tried to get some sleep in my own bed, then another bed. I tried falling asleep on the couch, the floor and other places, but I couldn't sleep. I began peeing in a cup so I could see if my pee had blood in it, and to catch any blood clots if I peed out any more. I had blood in my pee a few times that first week or two, but only peed blood clots that first night, then once more. I was doing everything I could think of to help myself, but nothing was really helping. It was tough to find anything to eat, because I had pretty much lost my appetite. About the only thing I could stand to eat was canned whole kernel corn.

So I ate corn every day and sipped a little tea until I couldn't stand to eat any more. Believe me, it wasn't much food. I never ate a whole can at one time. The best I ever felt for a moment or two here and there, was when I would do some sit ups with the new AB Chair I received the day after I pissed those first blood clots. I would do 2-3 hundred a day. Anything to lessen the discomfort and pain for even a moment here and there! Using that AB Chair was the only real relief I got until I drank some lemon balm tea.

After about a week or more had passed with me doing the same daily routine of trying to pee, trying to sleep and trying all kinds of things to feel better...I asked my wife if there was anything she could think of that we had NOT tried. While she was thinking about that I said "What about lemon balm tea?" Then I said "No, I don't see how that would help. But hey, let's try some anyway." Besides the lower back pain and other body aches, I even felt pain and discomfort from my crotch all the way to my throat the whole time. I had gotten use to all of it by the time I tried the lemon balm tea. My stomach ached the whole time too. My wife made me the cup of lemon balm tea and when I took the first drink, I could feel that lemon balm tea going down my throat, down my chest, hitting my stomach and beyond. Boy did that feel good.

At first I just thought that I was feeling the heat from the tea. But I actually started to feel better. I could hardly believe it! Then I got to thinking.... Maybe I just think I'm feeling better? Maybe I just want to think the lemon balm tea helped? But since it made me feel the best I had felt in almost two weeks, I drank two more cups that day and felt better after each cup. As I kept pissing into a clear glass cup, I noticed there wasn't blood in my pee. My pee wasn't pinkish like it had been the whole time those two weeks. So I kept drinking cups of lemon balm tea; at least 4 or 5 cups a day. I could hardly resist drinking it because I was so beat down, sick, hurting, aching, dazed, shocked, scared and as tired as I have ever been. I even began to think I was going to be OK, and even thought about canceling the doctor's appointment. But since I was far from being well, I kept that doctor's appointment.

Now, before I go on, let me tell you what my wife began to notice about my body. She noticed that I had about a dozen bruises on my back. As we both began to look for more bruises we found the most obvious bruise which was on my right side just below my ribs, bruises on my arms here and there and other places. There was about 15-20 bruises total. I wondered what the heck is going on? I haven't done anything to get all those bruises! So where'd they come from? What caused them? It was a few weeks before I finally realized what had caused them. My doctor's appointment is the next thing that happened. So, I'll tell you what caused those bruises when I get to the time I found out a few weeks later.

When I got to the doctor's office, which was a local well-known medical clinic a block from the hospital, the doctor didn't really know what was wrong with me exactly, so he did some tests. He did tell me that day that I had high blood pressure and he would give me something for that high blood pressure. As I was leaving, the doctor gave me some samples of the medication he thought I should take. When he handed me the medication I asked him "How long do I need to take this?" The doctor replied "The rest of your life." I was dumb founded immediately. Here I had been free of sickness for decades and the doctor was telling me I would have to take drugs for the rest of my life! Holy crap, I thought! I thought maybe when he gets my test results back he'll change his tune? I couldn't imagine being on drugs the rest of my life.

Everyone had made such a big deal about me being on drugs from age 19-26, that it was weird hearing anyone tell me I NEEDED to take drugs the rest of my life. I felt like I should have just stayed on drugs in the first place and never got off them. I couldn't handle the thought of doing drugs. So it took me a couple of days to actually start taking the drugs he had given me. I was taking Nisoldipine. It made me feel yucky. But I kept taking it anyway, since that's all I had. The doctor's office called the day after my appointment and told me that it looks like I have kidney disease and that I needed to come back in within the next two weeks. So as I waited to go back to the doctor, I took my Nisoldipine and continued drinking lemon balm tea and using my new AB Chair; working on trying to feel better.

My test results revealed that my creatinine was 2.9 and so was my potassium. Normal creatinine for a male is 1.5. Normal potassium level is between 3.6 and 5.2. So my creatinine proved I had kidney disease for at least 14 months prior to these tests; which would be about April 2005. My identical 2.9 potassium level was well below normal, so the doctor gave me a prescription for high potency potassium. This went a long ways in relieving the immense tension I had been feeling for the past 3 weeks. I went from being iron man to Gumby the rubber man. Once I had taken all of that prescription I felt better but still had nervous like tension. It wasn't something I had felt before my whole life. It turned out to be my blood pressure going as high as 240/140 a lot. While all this was going on with me I also had to deal with my mother being in the hospital on her death bed.

I went to my second doctor's appointment about the 25th of October and the doctor said he was scheduling 2 CAT scans for me to find out if I had kidney stones or anything else wrong in my lower torso. I told him that there was no way I could have kidney stones because I take magnesium regularly. But he insisted. So I went along. But when I went to the office that handled the scheduling for the CAT scans, I told them I would have to know how much it was going to cost before I could agree to them. I told them if they cost too much then I'll just have to do without them, if I couldn't afford them.

They had never had anyone ask them this. The lady called several people in the clinic. Then called the hospital that actually did the CAT scans, but no one could tell me the cost of the CAT scans. I told them I would have to know before I could agree to take the CAT scans. They said they would have to call me and let me know when they found out. I thought that was ridiculous! They called the next day and said it would be $1100, so I refused and said I guess I'll just have to die since I can't afford it. My next doctor's appointment was a few days before Christmas. But in the meantime, some very bad things happened and I was about to start what turned out to be what saved my life.

My mother had been in a nursing home for 20 months when she had to be rushed to the hospital and put on a ventilator to stay alive. Her heart had given out, mostly because she was 85 years old. This was almost a month later to the day after my kidneys failed around October 6, 2006. I was pretty sure this was the end for my mother, so my wife and I went to the hospital every day to stay with her as long as they would let us. One of those first days I was standing at the end of my mother's bed and my wife asked "Why are your lips so dark red?" I immediately wiped my finger across my lips and said "Oh no! That's blood." And sure enough my throat starting bleeding again like it did back in early summer for 16-18 straight hours. I got scared about this.

Cold and flu season was in full swing and the thought of me catching a cold was terrifying. Just a tiny cough had started both throat bleeding episodes. I made my wife go straight to the shower as soon as she walked in the door, to try and wash off any cold or flu germs she might have on her clothes or body; since her work brings her in direct contact with many people every day.

Now while my mother was in the hospital for those last 10 days of her life, I was talking to the head nurse there named Pat. My Aunt Lora May Talley had been her usual hateful self and had taken control over who could see my mother or get any information on her condition. So I was trying to find out how such a bizarre thing could happen. Pat was helping me get that situation corrected. They ended up putting me as the person to represent my own mother, and I put a password to keep Lora May out.

I was use to her hatefulness. But I just wasn't in the mood for it for obvious reasons. Lora May had given me a scolding speech a few days earlier about how the only thing to do was pull the plug and let my mother die. I was never going to do that. My only thoughts were to fight for her life. I am always in favor of Life. As Pat and I were talking about all this, I mentioned that I had just been diagnosed with chronic kidney disease.

We got to talking about this, and she told me her husband also had kidney disease. So I asked her what he was doing about it and did she know anything that could possibly help me. **Now what she was about to tell me didn't seem like it was all that important, but it's what she told me that led me to the information that I know saved my life, by arresting and reversing my chronic kidney disease.** She told me that what her husband was doing was taking ginger packs and putting them on his back where his kidneys are. **She said the ginger packs, poultice, draws the poisons out of his kidneys.** This is what led me to saving my own life. Did ginger packs save my life? No. I never got that far. But as soon as Pat told me this I was extremely excited.

This was the first thing I had heard that would help someone with chronic kidney disease. The doctors only gave me dialysis and death within 2-3 years. As I began looking for the ginger root to do exactly what Pat had told me about, **I asked myself the question that is the question that actually ended up saving my life - What if you never put the poisons IN your body? Then you wouldn't HAVE to get them out! So that's what I began to do and do so obsessively.** After all, 2-3 years to live doesn't give you any time to wait around for a cure or help. The only reason I valued what Pat told me was that it was the ONLY help I had gotten. So it was dialysis, death or ginger packs!

At the same time my mother passed away November 14 and that hit me hard. The day of her funeral it was around freezing with sleet and rain. So I couldn't even go to her funeral, since I couldn't risk exposing myself to weather that could give me a cold or the flu. Remember, my throat was bleeding and if I caught a cold, the coughing from that cold would keep my throat bleeding for days; enough to bleed to death. After my mom died, I dragged around in a daze, not caring much about how near death I was.

It was during those following days while I was wondering where the poisons came from that had made my kidneys fail, that I thought - I had eaten pretty healthy for decades, so this poisons idea wasn't making sense to me. It's right here where I realized some of the poisons I had overlooked were in those fruit juices I was drinking. I would get that wired up tense feeling after drinking juices. Then began to recognize that same feeling when I ate or drank other things. I didn't think they were poison at that time. I just didn't like that wired up tense feeling, no matter what was causing it. So I was getting serious about finding out what was causing that feeling.

I knew what I ate and drank to give me that feeling, but what was in those products that was THE cause of it? I began to form my own opinion, but didn't have any idea if I was right about the opinion I was forming. I was going to stick with my developing opinion until someone told me something better that would help me. As this opinion was just beginning I went for my 3rd doctor's appointment and my 2nd blood tests to see how my kidneys were doing.

My test results came back December 26 and revealed that my creatinine was going up point 1 a month and was now 3.1. My potassium was 5.7 after being 2.9 just 2 months ago. My BUN had gone up from 30 to 44 too. BUN is basic urea nitrogen, which basically is a sign of your kidney's inability to digest protein. As a result, my doctor insisted I should see Dr. Edwards, the clinic's nephrologist. But during that visit I was there over 2 hours. That's when they took my blood pressure and it was 240/140. I just sat there calmly and they were pretty frantic. The doctor said "Your blood pressure is dangerously high".

It was 240 over 140. So they started giving me Atenolol, and had me put in under my tongue. The nurse would come back in about 20 minutes and take my blood pressure, leave the room, come back and give me some more Atenolol to put under my tongue. We went through this routine at least 3 times and finally they said I could leave. I was given a prescription and told to see Dr. Edwards as soon as possible. I still had that nervous tension that high blood pressure gives you. I didn't know it at the time, but that Atenolol they gave me doesn't really lower blood pressure. It only slows your heart down so your high blood pressure doesn't do as much damage to your organs. So you can see that yucky Nisoldipine let my blood pressure rise to 240/140 or more. All the Atenolol was doing was slowing my heart down.

During that visit, Dr. Forte did something that shocked me. He had always been a quiet man and said very little to me for the most part. I had made it a point NOT to tell him about the lemon balm tea stopping my internal bleeding and giving me such significant relief over the past 3 months. But I ended up saying something about it and he raised his voice in a snap and yelled angrily "Well, did your lemon balm tea tell you you have chronic kidney disease?" I stayed silent to keep him from blowing up even worse. I had kept my mouth shut about it all along because I was worried about making someone mad if I mentioned it. I never mentioned anything like that to him again.

I did what the doctor and nurses told me to do and that included taking the Nisoldipine and the 100mg Atenolol daily. The 100mg Atenolol was only suppose to slow my heart down to about 60 beats a minute, but ended up slowing my heart to 40 BPM. So they had to lower that to 50mg Atenolol. I told them I was gonna stop taking the Nisoldipine, since it was yucky and costs quite a bit. It was gonna cost over $1000 a year. I was paying cash for everything. So, that cost was unreasonable to me and my cash. I worked with a nurse and we finally found a calcium channel blocker called Amlodipine for me to take, along with the 50mg Atenolol. But as December turned into January and into spring, I was busy doing everything I could do to help myself.

And what I was doing was researching on the INTERNET, trying to find anything that might help me and what those things were and did for you. This was kind of hard because my eyes had gotten bad all the sudden because of my kidney failure and high blood pressure. I had to find my mother's reading glasses and use them to read anything on the INTERNET or food labels. I had no idea what, if anything, was going to help me; since doctors only gave me dialysis, death, drugs, tests and high doctor bills. So I worked hard on finding poisons in my food, drinks and hygiene items and water.

I admit, I became obsessed. But all my life I've been the best at most things I do; football, baseball, track, faster runner, playing guitar and in bands and more. So I was gonna do the same about trying to save my own life and now, get rid of the poisons entering my body through my water, food, drinks and hygiene items. So as I waited for my appointment with Dr. Edwards, the clinic's nephrologist, I worked feverishly on this. Once I stopped drinking all the high fructose corn syrup soaked sodas and juices, I started feeling a lot better during these early months of 2007.

Besides starting my own personal war to eliminate high fructose corn syrup from my diet, I was doing lots and lots of other things too. We got our shower filter, then our fluoride water filter, stopped buying red meat, quit buying sugar, quit cooking with the microwave, changed to organic soaps, less toxic toothpaste and more; just in those first few months of all this. I realized it could all turn out to be a waste of time and money. But my money was no good to me dead. So I stuck with this obsession for the next few years.

Another obsession I quickly developed was taking my blood pressure! They recommended that I take it every day. But old obsession boy ME did it excessively. I took my blood pressure 30-40 times a day. I wanted to see what effect all kinds of activities and foods had on my blood pressure. But my actual blood pressure was taken following all the guidelines required to accurately take blood pressure, when I did it. They never follow these guidelines in the doctor's office or hospitals. So their results are near meaningless. My real blood pressure stayed about 160-180 over 90-110 the first 3 months of 2007, taking 50mg Atenolol and 10mg Amlodipine daily.

I was also working on my high potassium and had only my potassium tested every couple of weeks until my appointment with Dr. Edwards. When I finally got to that appointment with Dr. Edwards, a nephrologist, I was scared about seeing how much worse my kidneys were than back in December. I expected my creatinine to be up from 3.1 to at least 3.5 and bring me less than 2 years from having to go on dialysis.

When the day of my appointment came it was the first week of April and I was glad I was going to get some real help now. Dr. Edwards ordered more blood tests, a urinalysis and prescribed me Clonidine, to go along with the Amlodipine and Atenolol I was already taking. He also asked me to take my blood pressure every day and give him the results for the next two weeks once I had them. But in the meantime, my test results came back. I had some protein in my urine and my potassium was still high at 5.5, but everything else was normal...except my BUN and creatinine; which are the two factors doctors use to determine kidney function. My BUN had gone down from 44 in December to just 27 and my creatinine, instead of going up to 3.5 as the doctors said it would, went DOWN...all the way down to 2.6! That was a 9 month swing in my favor plus the last 4 months to boot! I couldn't believe it and really wasn't sure what had caused this human miracle, or if it would last!

I reported my daily blood pressure readings to Dr. Edwards two weeks later as he had asked for. My overall average blood pressure was 145/75 for the two weeks, but my pulse was just 55. So they said to come back and see Dr. Edwards in a year. But in the meantime, I continued to see Dr. Forte and talk to one male nurse named Matt. I didn't like the idea of being tied to doctors, so I didn't go back for 6 months. I don't have records covering this one year from mid April 2007 until March 2008.

One bizarre thing did happen during this time. When I went back to see Dr. Forte, some female nurse was doing the usual line of questions and I was answering them as I always did. But then she asks "Do you believe you have chronic kidney disease?" I hesitated, and smiled, thinking…is this a real question or a trick question? Since the doctors said that I did, I thought it was settled. I answered her and said "That's what the doctors say." She then typed for a minute or so into her laptop. I later found out she had not recorded what I actually said. She put in my medical records that I did not believe I had chronic kidney disease, and that I believed I could heal myself of my chronic kidney disease. I only found out because I allowed DHS to look at my medical records in an effort to get some help paying for the expensive drugs I had to take.

They wanted me to go see a psychiatrist. I was as puzzled as I could be. And even more so since it wasn't standard procedure. So I demanded a copy of my medical records from the clinic I was going to. I read through my medical records and that's how I found out about this.

Hey! Sure I'm crazy IF I think I can cure myself of a disease that I don't even believe I have, according to Nurse Fibber! LOL Problem was…I never even thought such a thing, much less SAID it. I realized she had asked the question because I had said I was going to be cured. But that was only because I had not accepted what they said about no one ever being cured or getting better with chronic kidney disease. And all I cared about was being cured and well. I didn't realize yet that I was never going to get any help for my kidneys at that clinic or from those doctors.

But the next time I went back to the doctor after seeing that garbage on my medical records I spoke to Nurse Fibber about what she wrote. She insisted that she only wrote what I said. Bah hum bug! When the only nurse that had helped me stepped in, he explained that they can't remove anything from my medical records, but they can put a note saying the patient never actually said that. So I dropped it.

During that year from April 2007 to March 2008, I kept doing the drugs for high blood pressure; since they said if I didn't, my kidneys would get worse even faster than they have so far. But I worked on getting rid of the poisons in my food, drinks and personal hygiene items. Remember, once I got the fluoride water filter and the shower filter in early 2007, my water was pure and safe; except for about 10% of the chlorine and all the fluoride in the shower water. So I worked on avoiding the poisons in our food, drinks and hygiene items and drank at least 3 quarts of water a day. I also drank Goji, Mangosteen and Noni juice a lot. I ate lots of fruits and vegetables, fish, chicken and turkey, but no red meat or pork to speak of. I was getting depressed from time to time because the doctors had done nothing for my kidneys; only for the high blood pressure that caused the chronic kidney disease.

You gotta remember…my mother had been in a nursing home for the past 21 months, then died the month after I was diagnosed with chronic kidney disease. My mother had to file for bankruptcy because Regions Bank would not take payments from me when my mother became unable to care for herself at all; as though this kinda thing was unheard of to Regions Bank. We barely saved the house from auction 9 months before my mom passed. All the doctors said I would be dead or on dialysis by 2008 and no later than 2009.

There was no hope for any future for me and I was all on my own to save my own life without any real help from anybody. You talk about pressure! I just want you to know what I went through while I was saving my own life, without knowing that I was. Who was I to say doctors were wrong? I was a dying man with just a couple of years left to live. I kept on taking my blood pressure a few dozen times a day all the way up until my next and second visit to Dr. Edwards in March 2008.

I had gotten to where when I went to the doctor I would ask "Is this the visit where you finally help me with my kidneys?" But that day never came. When I went to see Dr. Edwards the second time it was kinda awkward. I asked him about doing herbal cleanses and taking herbs. He said he had never studied herbs. Now if you know herbs are medicine, which they are, then you know Dr. Edwards told me that he had never studied medicine; which is actually true.

Seriously. I also had him take a look at my nipples. Yea, my manly nipples! I was actually growing tits, and was shocked at what was happening. They were just beginning to swell up. Dr. Edwards said that I had low testosterone and prescribed me Viagra. That took care of a symptom, but not the real problem, low testosterone. He also called for blood tests to test my kidney function again and to test me for PTH, parathyroid hormone levels. The tests came back showing my PTH levels were high. But my CMP, complete metabolic, results on March 31, 2008 shocked me. My creatinine had gone down from 2.6 in April 2007 to 2.2.

Remember, my creatinine was 3.1 on December 26, 2006. So instead of my creatinine being 4.6 in March 2008 as doctors insisted it would be, my creatinine was down to 2.2. I had added 24 months to my life already. Wow!

How did that happen? My potassium was also down to 4.1 compared to 5.5 a year earlier, and marked the first time my potassium had been in the normal range since my kidneys failed over 18 months earlier.

When the nurse called me to give me the results, she said I needed to take some new drug called something like Calcitril. She said Dr. Edwards was prescribing it to bring down my PTH levels. I said OK, but wanted to make sure there wasn't anything natural to help before I agree to any more drugs. I called the nurse back a few days later and discussed the possibility of taking calcium supplements instead of the drug. She was against that, but said she would ask the doctor and get back to me. See, your PTH levels rise if your body's parathyroid glands detect low calcium levels in your blood. Problem was, that my calcium was always mid-range normal. And also, the Amlodipine I was taking was a calcium channel blocker. It was blocking calcium from getting into my heart to keep my heart from retracting as hard, thus lowering my blood pressure. In other words, the Amlodipine was the cause of the high PTH levels. So I decided to find a way to stop taking the Amlodipine to solve this problem by eliminating the cause.

Now, since most of you probably don't know. A person with chronic kidney disease gets worse progressively. Your creatinine increases and your skin itches more and more because of it. You lose your appetite. You become anemic. Your ankles, face and other places get swollen because your kidneys aren't removing fluids from your body properly. And your metabolics get more and more out of whack until this and the skin itching can only be relieved by dialysis. You also grow closer and closer to becoming a diabetic and almost always do. So I had to work on preventing diabetes too.

When I called the clinic to find out why I hadn't heard from the nurse about that PTH thing, they wouldn't talk to me and made excuses. I was trying also to see when Dr. Edwards wanted me to come back to see him. But the end of May I received 2 certified letters from both of my doctors at that clinic. They both said that within 30 days they would no longer be my doctors and that they would forward my medical records to the doctor of my choice. Dr. Edwards stated that this action was "due to non-compliance and general resistance to his recommendations for your care." That pissed me off and shocked me at first. It was ridiculous though because I had done everything they told me to do except for jumping right on that last drug Dr. Edwards had wanted me to take. Asking questions isn't resistance. Seeking alternatives isn't either. So it became clear to me that it had to be over me getting better by doing things for myself, while they demonstrated their helpless and unwilling interest in my health; much less helping me get better.

But I called them and tried to talk to them, and they were mean and hateful and belligerent. I was calling to ask when I could come and pick up 2 of my prescriptions that came straight from the manufacturer to the doctor's office, and to get my other prescriptions to be refilled. But they refused and told me not to call again or they would have me arrested. So I dropped it and never talked to them again. I did talk to a wonderful person I had become friends with in the business office, Carolyn. She let me talk to her about paying Clopton Clinic the money I still owed them; which I paid in full with cash. So for all of June, July and 12 days of August I had no doctor or prescriptions and was all by myself again trying to save my own life.

I heard there was a free church clinic in the old Holiday Inn building down town. So I gave them a call and learned I qualified to come there. My appointment was for August 12, 2008. When I got there for my appointment I was surprised to see that a girl friend, not girlfriend, was working there. So, I talked with her about when we were in high school, who she married and if she had any kids; and of course, about my visit there. Everybody was real nice to me and my visit went real well. It was pretty uneventful. But at least I had a doctor again, after being thrown out of Clopton Clinic for getting better. I did have my blood tested and the results came back a couple of days later. My potassium was just 4.3. My BUN had dropped to 24 and my creatinine was 2.37; which was slightly above my last result of 2.1 five months earlier. I was relieved to find this out. I scheduled my next appointment for September. But a few days after my first appointment I made a surprise discovery.

I had been searching the INTERNET for almost two years for a cure for my chronic kidney disease, but hadn't found one. Actually, I hadn't even come close to finding a cure. I hadn't even found anyone claiming to cure kidney disease. All I had found so far was a book by a great pioneering doctor from John Hopkins Medical Center who had done clinical trials limiting his patients to 20 grams of protein daily to slow down the progression of kidney disease. His name was Mackenzie Walser. I had found his book titled "Coping With Kidney Disease – A 12-Step Treatment Program to Help You Avoid Dialysis", and I ordered it from Amazon.com. What Dr. Walser had done is develop a program based on a British program that was a no protein diet. Dr. Walser's program was based on a 20 grams of protein daily diet.

I read the book and started to follow his program. I had trouble sticking with the 20 grams of protein daily. But I worked on limiting my protein, but could never get by with just 20 grams of protein daily. I had been working on this for over a year by the time I had my first appointment at the church health clinic. My tests results proved Dr. Walser's program was helping me because my BUN was down to 24.

After my first appointment on August 12, 2008, I was searching the INTERNET for the part of the title of Dr. Walser's book "avoiding dialysis". Much to my surprise, there was a new search result besides Dr. Walser's book. It was for GenoMed. I read over the site and saw they claimed to have superior clinical outcomes for several chronic conditions which included kidney disease caused by hypertension. I figured I could debunk that garbage quickly. So while I was reading over the web site, I found an email address I could contact them about participating in their superior clinical outcome program. I knew I was gonna get some dumb reply about worshiping the doctor while I paid him huge amounts of money in my quest to save my life. I had emailed the top dog at GenoMed, Dr. David Moskowitz on August 21; just 9 days after my first appointment at the church clinic. Dr. Moskowitz said he could help me; but that we needed to act quickly since my creatinine was currently 2.37.

By the fourth email, Dr. Moskowitz had laid out what I needed and told me to give the information to my doctor at the church clinic, Dr. Pyle. I didn't really understand the program at this time, but took the information with me at my next appointment at the church clinic. But before I got to my appointment, I received notice that I had been approved for Medicaid. I had applied almost 18 months ago to get some help paying my $300+ monthly drug bill. DHS told me repeatedly that the only way I could get that kind of help was to apply for Medicaid. They wanted me to apply for Food Stamps, but that was ridiculous. I only needed some help with that high monthly drug bill! As a result of me receiving approval for Medicaid, I no longer qualified for the church health clinic. So when I went for my second and last appointment there, I told them I couldn't come back any more.

While I was there, Dr. Pyle and I talked about what I needed for his program, but Dr. Pyle explained how he couldn't start me on the drugs Dr. Moskowitz ordered, since Dr. Pyle could not be my doctor any more. But Dr. Pyle did try to get me in to see a doctor who was a friend of his, Dr. Henry Allen. As we were talking, Dr. Pyle happened to mention how he and his friends use to come out to the fairgrounds and watch us play baseball. I said "Really? Who were you going out there to watch?" Dr. Pyle said "You. You were the best player. We went out there to see you." I was pleasantly surprised and told him "Gee thanks Dr. Pyle. Glad you enjoyed watching me play." I was surprised because all I had heard from the doctors was one asshole thing after another without any real sign of any doctor caring one damned bit!

Dr. Pyle said all he could do is give me a prescription for one drug Dr. Moskowitz suggested, since he wouldn't need to monitor me for that drug. I thanked Dr. Pyle and told him and his staff that I was sad that I couldn't come back, and that I wished the greatest success for the wonderful service they were providing. So there I was, back to square one with no doctor. But with Medicaid approved for me then, I felt pretty good about finding a new doctor.

I contacted Dr. Allen's office which was White River Rural Health Clinic at that time. After talking to several employees there, they got all confused about what I had discussed with Dr. Pyle about what Dr. Moskowitz ordered for me. So they said they couldn't help me. I had DHS send me a complete list of doctors in my area who accepted Medicaid. I went through the whole list and after contacting 45 doctors I had been turned down by each and every one of them. They didn't want ANYTHING to do with someone getting cured, and it didn't matter how offensive that was coming from all those doctors and staffs. It made it even more offensive after being kicked out of Clopton Clinic for getting better! I kept in contact with Dr. Moskowitz during September, October and November, always explaining how no doctor would go along with any plan to cure people or help them get better.

But toward the end of November I decided to call Dr. Pyle back. Dr. Pyle's real job is as Vice President of our main hospital. He volunteered at the church health clinic to work for free. So I contacted him at the hospital.

Dr. Pyle was so kind to me. He said "Well, let me give them a call and see what I can do." I thought...Dr. Pyle had already done that and it didn't work out, so it's not gonna work this time either. But much to my surprise, White River Rural Health Clinic called me and asked for some personal information and made me an appointment as Dr. Pyle had asked them to do.

The appointment was for December 4. I contacted Dr. Moskowitz and told him the good news and he instructed me as to what I needed to tell the doctor. My visit with Dr. Allen went well and he prescribed the medications Dr. Moskowitz had ordered for me, and I began taking them on December 8. Gee! So my six month ordeal since being thrown out of Clopton Clinic for getting better seemed to be over.

I figured I would get thrown out of White River Rural Health Clinic too. I hadn't had too much respect for doctors since becoming an adult and the bizarre backwards treatment and attitudes of Dr. Edwards and Forte had only made that worse and darker. But I kept thinking about friends of mine who are doctors and kept some positive hope because of them. I couldn't even imagine my dear friend Lance Rainey not caring about people. All I knew about him was as good as it gets.

Lance and I were in our first band together when I was 14 years old, and that band was the most popular band of our age group for 4 years. We were like brothers until he had to go away to medical school. Lance's dad was also a doctor and helped me for free several times. I still love Lance, Dr. Lance Rainey that is. So don't think I am prejudice against doctors just because the facts about them are negative most of the time. I had reserved myself to going along with doctors and keeping my mouth shut about natural things to them.

After all, as much cash as I had to pay for whatever doctors did, I wasn't about to reject them to their faces or impede them from giving me information or aid. I was just a helpless dying man who doctors only forecast for my future was death, dialysis or kidney transplant. All I cared about was saving my own life. There had been no light at the end of the tunnel for me among doctors and the medical profession. That was about to all change. Two doctors joined my team, the Life team, the results matter team, the CURES are acceptable team, the Your Health now matters team...and maybe the Liars Can Now Eat Their Own poopie team! Ha ha!

I was now starting Dr. Moskowitz's program and since this was a doctor who had already proven his treatments work through his work in clinical trials, I wouldn't have to listen to so many people tell me how crazy I am about this doctor's treatment; like so many people have done about my gospel of poisons saturating our entire food, drinks and water supplies. Also, I had to sign a non-disclosure agreement agreeing not to talk about the specifics of his patented treatments and clinical trials. But Dr. Moskowitz has given me specific permission as to what I CAN tell you. So I must stick to that agreement, and those of you reading this will have to excuse me for being vague about this for this reason. Please.

After I had started the treatment on December 8, I went back to Dr. Allen's office to get my blood tested on the 15th. I had to do this while we were upping the dose of the medication as Dr. Moskowitz advised. Those tests showed my creatinine was 2.2 and my potassium was 4.1. We were trying to see if the treatment was causing a rise in either one. Since all was good, we upped the dose. Next blood test was January 8. My creatinine was 2.13 and potassium was 4.3. No problem. So we upped the dose again. Next test was January 30. My creatinine was 2.15 and my potassium was 4.4. So no problem and we upped the dose again.

Next test was February 17. My creatinine was down to 2.0 and my potassium was 4.6. So, like always, we upped the dose. Next test was March 9th. I was shocked to see that my creatinine was all the way down to 1.9! My potassium was 4.6. So it was clear to me that this treatment was really working. But since the time I started this treatment on December 8, 2008 up until the second week of March 2009, I had been laying off the other drugs almost entirely. It was extremely difficult for me to get the drug I needed for this treatment. I had to get a new prescription almost every time we upped the dose, and I had to find where to get it for a good price.

Paying $300+ a month just for this one drug was going to be a long term problem as far as I could see. Medicaid wouldn't pay a penny for that particular drug. It's not on their list. Do wah diddie diddie dumb dumb dumb! But there was nothing I could do except keep on paying cash. Another problem during all these tests and upping the dose, was my blood pressure had gone up to 203/135! Yikes.

See, Dr. Moskowitz said there was chance, not a certainty, that I might be able to just end up on the one drug he was using to arrest my kidney disease. I was and still am against doing drugs. So I stay obsessed with doing as little drugs as I think I can get away with. What I do end up taking doesn't bother me though. I think about all those ibuprofen, aspirin, Aleve, Tylenol and antacids I do NOT take any more. So my drug intake is actually LESS than what it was the past 20 years.

With my blood pressure at 203/135, I didn't flip out or even get scared. I was just pissed because I knew I would have to get back to taking those other drugs along with the high doses of the drug at the center of my treatment. I didn't take my blood pressure again, because I knew my anger only made it go even higher. I did contact Dr. Moskowitz to see what he recommended. But it was only an improved version of what all I had been taking. None the less, we were both glad my creatinine was down to 1.9 and I had reached the dosage I needed to be on. What I already came to know was that, all you can do about high blood pressure is take more drugs if your blood pressure is high. Doctors sure don't have a cure for high blood pressure. I'm working on that for myself, but think it was probably caused by gene mutation or DNA damage from high fructose corn syrup.

I went to work to find a way to get that one drug cheaper. I found a lot of places online that claimed they could help. I spent quite a bit of time reading all the terms and services available for discount drugs. The best one seemed to be RX OutReach. And it was in the same city Dr. Moskowitz was in and one of my favorite cities too. RX OutReach, www.rxoutreach.org, allows you to buy a 90 day supply of one medication for $20 and $55 for a 180 day supply. It doesn't matter the dosage or the frequency of the dose either. So even though my prescribed dosage for my main drug is 6x the normal dose, I still get it for those same prices.

I did have a problem at the very first because their pharmacy rejected my order because of the unusual high dosage. I gave a desperate plea to them to fill my order. They still refused. But I had my doctor send them a fax and got it all cleared up. So I got my order a few days after that. I tell ya. Something was always popping up as an obstacle to me trying to get well, no matter who, what, when or where I made the effort to get help from the medical profession!

Once I got all this tangled mess worked out about trying to get all the drugs I now needed because of that one main drug, getting back on the drugs I had backed off after starting the treatment, getting a local doctor to help with all this and a few other lesser problems, I felt I was in the best shape yet. But when I had my next blood test April 13, my creatinine had gone UP to 2.3 from

1.9 just five weeks earlier! I thought, oh my God, I've really messed up now! I was shattered. I thought the worst. After all, there had never been any real hope for getting well. So I wasn't really surprised; just defeated in my quest to cure myself or at least never have to be on dialysis.

I figured that my blood pressure going up to 203/135 and probably being up for a few weeks, caused damage to my kidneys as the explanation for my creatinine going up from 1.9 to 2.3 in just 5 weeks! That was 4x the rate of creatinine rising from kidney failure you are supposed to have. So I was scared as I waited for my next tests I insisted on just 3 weeks later. On May 4 my creatinine was holding at 2.3. BUN was 24 and potassium was 4.5. This dumb founded me and neither Dr. Allen nor Dr. Moskowitz could explain what had or was happening. I had my theory, but couldn't be for sure. But my next test about 2 months later, July 31, showed my creatinine was still holding at 2.3. But there was no sign that my kidneys had actually gotten worse. I thought about this until sometime in the fall and finally concluded that my creatinine had gone down to 1.9, then back up to 2.3 in five weeks because I had gone back to taking Atenolol which slowed my heart down by about 1/3.

I concluded this as THE cause, and realized that slowing my heart down made a point 3 difference, and that there had been no further damage to my kidneys, much less...major damage. Then when I got my test results for December 10, I was convinced of this and breathed a big sigh of relief. I also breathed a GIGANTIC sigh of relief because I was still alive at the end of 2009, and was not on dialysis either, as all the doctors insisted I would be! Now all I had to do was to maintain what I had achieved.

Back in June I had kinda fallen off the horse about avoiding high fructose corn syrup. I could barely say anything about it without people being totally disinterested and downright hateful a lot of times, and crazy. So I gave up on that and started back not caring how much high fructose corn syrup I consumed. This went on for June, July and into August when I woke up with gout one morning in August 2009. I said oh no. I hope this goes away soon. It hurt so horrifyingly bad. So I stopped chugging down the high fructose corn syrup and ate extremely well again.

But that gout stayed with me for TWO WHOLE MONTHS. I yelled and screamed a lot and laid down most of the time. I was in such miserable pain that I couldn't even imagine how I could get to a doctor. Shoot...the 15 foot trip to the bathroom was filled with mind numbing pain, yelling and screaming and the horror of having to make that same trip back to the bed or lounger!

It was during this two month long affliction of gout that sealed the doom for high fructose corn syrup with me forever. And I mean FOREVER! I thought there might be another episode of gout even after I got off the high fructose corn syrup, to prove me wrong. But it never came. And I have not had any gout since. The doctor gave me some pills to take if I think gout is coming on; which I have used twice, but never did have gout. I took it as a precaution two times.

Another situation that was going on for most of this time was DHS fighting against me to keep me from getting what was lawfully and legally mine. Remember, I applied for Medicaid to get some help paying my $300+ monthly drug bill. Before I applied, I checked to see if I had a chance of qualifying. The terms state that if your disease is expected to last more than 12 months or end in death, then you qualify. And since doctors all claimed that all chronic kidney patients end up dead and their disease lasts more than 12 months, I knew I qualified. The word chronic clarifies that! But the phony government works AGAINST the People, not FOR the People. So I had to fight them for 18 months. Fortunately for me, I knew I qualified. So no matter what corrupt behavior DHS used, I knew to let it go and keep appealing.

Their goal is to force you to fight them on your death bed to get what is legally and lawfully yours! They hope to at least delay you from getting anything in hopes you will go ahead and die to avoid you getting what is legally and lawfully yours! This vile anti-American behavior should not be tolerated in America.

As 2009 ended and 2010 began, I decided I was going back to living my life after this 5 year ordeal of huge ups and downs with my life in the balance. I felt like I had kept my kidney disease in check and improved greatly. Just the fact that I went from 3.1 creatinine in December 2006 to 2.1 in December 2009 was incredible, and unheard of in the medical profession any way! My creatinine should've been 5.7 at that time, but was only 2.1! So I had already added SIX YEARS to my life. Three years I had not gotten worse, plus the three years it would take for me to need dialysis if I started getting worse after December 2009! And I had learned to control my potassium.

And all that time I never developed any further symptoms of chronic kidney disease. I didn't get diabetes as they said I would either.

As a matter of fact, I had cured myself of headaches, heartburn, arthritis, dandruff, skin burns and itching and other things. But all I set out to do was save my own life by trying to cure myself of chronic kidney disease. I had all those other conditions and diseases for 20 years, and I had never thought about dying from them. It was the chronic kidney disease that brought all the death and end of my life talk.

I had talked to our local newspaper and TV station about doing a story to save a lot of lives. But they claimed I hadn't done what I had done, and that I couldn't claim I had since the medical profession didn't do it for me. It didn't even matter that three doctors had played a role in it. They weren't reporting any cures! I thought how sick that really was. But wasn't surprised at their rejection of reporting anything that would save lives or suffering. All they care about is reporting what big business does. They'll report the wonderful story of a child OR adult that doctors "cured", but was back in remission and about to die, and the new technology the medical profession buys to diagnose things better. But none of that will cure you.

I didn't try to talk them in to caring about people's lives. They made it more than clear that they would never even consider reporting anything that wasn't invented or done by the medical profession. **So, me being the only kidney patient in the area and being one of the rare rare ones in the entire country to arrest their kidney disease, was entirely meaningless and really offensive to them; our wonderful media!** Gag, hiccup, vomit!

This is where I decided to write this book. But I didn't because I really didn't think anyone would really be interested in their own life or health. Everyone insists on letting the doctors hold their hands and lead them to the grave to maximize doctors' income and never think there's any other way. It's sad, and even sadder that this dependency on doctors, instead of GOD and Nature, is perpetuated by christianity. I realized that even though the only hope tens of millions of people have for being healthy or being cured of disease is OUTSIDE the medical profession and christianity. But since everyone is fooled and too scared because of that deceit, no one was going to care about saving their own lives and the lives of their loved ones. So I decided not to waste my time writing this book. I wanted to go ahead and write this book, but the only thing people in this country believe is lies. So I didn't!

I had proved the doctors wrong by living beyond 2009 and not going on dialysis. And I was determined to go ahead and go back to living my life without death hanging over my head and being my ONLY possible future according to the medical profession. I was still searching for a cure, but continuing Dr. Moskowitz's treatment program and following my own ways that reversed my kidney disease. I was still trying to figure out what I had done that helped, from anything that actually didn't help me at all. And I was still all alone on this. I mean, who COULD I talk to that could tell me how a chronic kidney patient COULD get better or be cured?

I kept making regular searches on the INTERNET for this very thing; just as I had been doing since October 2006 when my kidneys failed. I thought I had found a cure when I ran across an advertisement on the INTERNET claiming an Australian man had cures, plural, for various kinds of chronic kidney disease. I was skeptical from the first. But at least he was saying what I wanted to hear...cures for kidney disease. So I forked out about $60 and bought his book and additional materials.

As I got to reading his book, I found many familiar things in his book. All of it was natural things, and that was exactly what I believed in. I gathered the information to start his "cure" for my chronic kidney disease caused by hypertension. The cure instructed me to take vitamins and herbs that I was already taking, but in different doses. The main adjustment I had to make was taking 600mg of Alpha Lipoic Acid. So I ordered the Alpha Lipoic Acid in the 600mg size and begin to take it and the other items in his so-called cure.

I told my doctor, Dr. Allen, and he cautioned me not to take the 600mg Alpha Lipoic Acid. I told him I was going to go ahead and take it, since no one else had any ideas how to cure me. But I agreed to only take it for 3-4 months, even though the "cure" called for me to take 600mg Alpha Lipoic Acid until I was cured. I took my blood tests during that doctor's visit on February 10, 2010. My creatinine was down to 1.9 and my potassium was 4.7. So I was ready to use this Australian man's "cure" to knock my kidney disease on out! I followed his "cure" until May 11.

When I went back to the doctor on May 11 I had my blood tested as I almost always did. My creatinine had gone UP to 2.2 and my potassium was 5.5! Yikes! That was the first time my potassium was out of the normal range in over three years. I was sure that I had messed up bad! But Dr. Allen told me that was exactly why he cautioned me about taking the 600mg Alpha Lipoic Acid. I knew Alpha Lipoic Acid caused your kidneys to reuse antioxidants, but never knew it did the same thing for potassium and other vitamins and minerals. So there I was, back in trouble again without knowing what was going on. And it was pretty clear that this Australian guy's alleged "cure" was not a cure at all. I admit that it could help those who knew practically nothing, but didn't really add anything to what I was already doing.

As a matter of fact, this guy discredits himself by not cautioning you on the grave dangers that his "cures" cause. If your potassium climbs to 6.0 or above, your heart will start to palpitate and it won't stop palpitating without emergency treatment. And there is nothing you can do to lower your potassium in a few minutes, hours or even days. So, his "cure" is quite dangerous and put my life in danger. Now I had to find a way to get my potassium down and keep it from going any higher. I thought this guy's "cure" might have even damaged my kidneys. I was scared and on edge from time to time for the weeks following this blood test and wondered if I was going to get better or worse. So I scheduled more blood tests 6 weeks later on June 23.

My test results for June 23, 2010 revealed that my creatinine went up from 2.2 to 2.3. The HUGE surprise was that my potassium had gone DOWN from 5.5 to 4.7! I was shocked and Dr. Allen was too, but not as much as I was. That's when he told me that was what he had cautioned me about the 600mg Alpha Lipoic Acid daily for. I thought that was really neat! But I told Dr. Allen right then and there that I had stopped taking the Alpha Lipoic Acid and that I was going to stop taking vitamins and herbs for at least a while.

After that, I felt I was at the end of my health improving and I was back on course heading back to dialysis and death; since my creatinine had gone up point 1 each and every month for the last four months; having gone up from 1.9 in February to 2.3 in May. So I decided to give up and go ahead and live what little life I had left. I took another six month break from doctors and accepted that I was getting worse and dreaded ever going back to the doctor. I just didn't want to know that my kidneys were getting progressively worse, so I stayed away. I finally got the courage to go back to the doctor after Thanksgiving and made an appointment for December 21. I dreaded what my blood tests were going to be.

The next day the doctor's office called and said my creatinine was 1.8. I was so relieved, but only for a few seconds, when they told me my potassium was 7.0! 7.0! Oh my GOD. I can die any time now! I started shaking real bad. I was so terrified. I kept saying "How could it be 7.0?" I haven't eaten any differently than I have been for the past 4 years. Then I thought…Oh no, my kidneys must be going bad in a hurry! But that didn't make any sense since my creatinine was only 1.8 and all my other metabolics were normal, except my BUN as usual. I didn't have time to think about it then. My life was on the line and I could die at any moment from the 7.0 potassium.

Finally, they told me I would need to go to the Emergency Room and have them put me on some inter-venous drug to bring my potassium level down. My wife and I got ourselves ready to go to the hospital and as bad as I hated going to the hospital, I went because there was no other way to save my life. They said they would let the hospital know I was on my way.

When we arrived, they told us to park by the emergency room thankfully. We rushed in and told them who I was. The girl I talked to after giving another woman my insurance information, said she needed to take my blood pressure. I said "You're not taking my blood pressure! You want to kill me? You take my blood pressure and it's going to scared the f*#king crap out of me and make my blood pressure go through the roof!" She just said "OK. I'll take it and won't tell you what it is." I replied "OK, but don't you dare tell me what it is. It doesn't matter any way."

After that, they led me to one of those little rooms beside the doctor and nurses station in the ER and had me lay on the table while my wife took a seat next to me. They immediately began to hook all these wires to me to monitor my blood pressure and pulse and my heart. I had to explain to them that even though I have chronic kidney disease, that they needed to realize that I am NOT like all the other kidney patients. I explained that I didn't have any symptoms of chronic kidney disease besides high blood pressure and elevated BUN and creatinine. Well, that is, besides the 7.0 potassium level I rushed to the ER about. I laid there on the bed, patient table, the whole time I was there for about 3 hours.

They took blood and urine to test, but were becoming obsessed and distracted by how high my blood pressure was. It was about 220/120 when I first came in. But the first time I knew about it, my blood pressure was 188/110. They were obsessed with this, but I wasn't bothered about it at all. Your blood pressure goes way up when you are scared or under stress. And I was BOTH, brother! I had feared my potassium going up like this for the past FOUR years and now that time had come. So all that fear over those four years took control of me once I was told by the doctor's office that my potassium was 7.0! While we were waiting on them to tell me the test results, my wife and I discussed what was going on and tried to figure out why my potassium was 7.0. After a while I told my wife that if I had to choose, I would say that the test result was wrong somehow, even though I had never had any test results that were wrong. Now if my creatinine had've been 2.9 or 3.0, I would've known my kidneys were getting worse and that was the problem. As I laid there, these young nurses kept coming in the room for various reasons.

When one of them asked me for my urine sample I said "Hey, couldn't we have some dinner BEFORE you ask me for my urine?" She got the joke and laughed and smiled as she left the room. When she came back, I asked how long it would be before my test results come back? She said about 45 minutes. They started in on my blood pressure again and gave me 0.2mg Clonidine for it to put under my tongue, as a faster way into my blood stream.

One time when she came in the room I looked at her and said "I became the only kidney patient in this area to ever get better. I had to do it myself. Doctors have no cures." She looked at me real funny and said "What?" I said "doctors have no cures", again. She said "Why do you say that?" I said "Well, if doctors have a cure for kidney disease, then tell me what it is right now. I want it!" "And by the way, if you have a cure for diabetes I'll take that right now too just as a precaution." She said "There isn't a cure for kidney disease or diabetes." And I replied "Didn't I just say that?" She smiled and said "Oh, I see why you said that." I said "Yea, because those are the facts. I wish it WASN'T though. I'd much rather be cured than to be right." Shortly after that the ER doctor came in the room.

When he entered my little ER room, the doctor said "Hello Mr. Cooksey. I'm Dr. Allen." I immediately said "No you're not. My doctor is Dr. Allen." He then said "I'm Dr. Allen. There are 3 Dr. Allens in town". I just laughed and let it go. He then began to tell me that my blood test came back and my potassium was just 4.8. I shouted out "I knew it!" And Dr. Allen continued. He said he was real worried about my blood pressure and that I needed to do this and that.

But I really didn't care, since I was only there because of the 7.0 potassium. I just wanted out of there. I didn't want to go in the first place. But I told Dr. Allen, Robert I think, that he could do whatever he felt he needed to do to satisfy himself as a doctor before I left. So he gave me some more Clonidine to put under my tongue. I laid there impatiently for about an hour and finally told a nurse that if they didn't take all those wires and IV off me, I was going to do it myself so I could leave. In about 10 minutes or so, they took all the stuff off me, gave me some orders to follow and let me go.

Now as I was leaving, I started thinking about what had just happened. I rushed to the hospital in fear of my life. Ran up a few thousand dollars in medical bills. And did so all because of an errant test result! I was as pissed as I was relieved! I called Dr. Pyle at the hospital and discussed the whole event. I told him I was almost scared to death literally and now had a multi-thousand dollar hospital bill, all because of a wrong test result that came from the hospital's lab in the first place. Dr. Pyle was once again the great reasonable man he had always proven himself to be, and said he would see to it that I didn't get a bill for any of this. I talked to him about what had caused the false test result and how it might be prevented in the future, as well as coming up with some type of protocol to handle this situation in the future.

Dr. Pyle wanted the same thing and said he would get something done about this for the future. I told Dr. Pyle that if I ever have a weird test result like that again, I would ignore it temporarily and go straight back to the doctor's office to give blood for another test. Then, and only then, would I accept the results as valid. He said that was a great idea. I thanked Dr. Pyle and said good bye. I never got a bill. Thank you Dr. Pyle. And that brings us to the end of the story up to now. I went back to the doctor on February 17, 2011 and will be going back in June for my next blood tests.

But as far as being scared or worried about my kidneys getting worse and having a relapse or worrying about anything bad happening to me medically, that is pretty much all behind me. I'm more worried about getting hit by a bus or being swept away in a tornado than I am of dying of chronic kidney disease now! But there are some things of importance I didn't get to while I was writing this chapter and going through my incredible journey with the medical profession and through the long line of poisons saturating our food, drinks and water supplies. Let me get to that now.

Remember when I told you about how I started growing tits. (Quit laughing.) It was traumatic. Ha ha! I was just worried about reversing that condition. It was caused by a high pressure medication; which impaired my body from producing enough testosterone. You can get this condition from eating chicken obsessively. I'm sure my chicken eating habits contributed to this condition, but the high blood pressure medication was almost all the cause.

Chicken has varying amounts of estrogen, which is basically female testosterone. The more estrogen in your body, the more female-ish your body gets. The doctor had wanted to prescribe me some testosterone cream or get an injection of testosterone from time to time. He also prescribed me Viagra. It sure did the job for the temporary impotence, but I was greatly impressed at how great it was for lowering my blood pressure. But at $13 a dose, I could hardly afford to take it very much.

So that fact and my tendency to find natural solutions finally led me to an herb called Tribulus Terrestris. Tribulus Terrestris does not create testosterone. What it does is cause production of the luteinizing protein (LH), which increases the natural production of testosterone. I took 2 250mg capsules of Tribulus Terrestris twice a day and in about 3 weeks I could tell those little tits of mine were going away. They were really hard knots under my nipples. I was really amazed. Another natural cure had worked for me. After a few more weeks, I didn't need the Viagra at all. But I wished I could afford it for high blood pressure. Luckily for me, I had just received those certified letters from my 2 doctors telling me they would no longer be my doctors. So I never told any doctor about how I had cured myself of those tits and temporary erectile dysfunction. You had better be thankful for what I've shared with you on this, because it IS a little embarrassing! But since it's a proven cure, I felt I must do so.

One other thing I did that really helped my kidneys was to take a product called Kidney Well; which is called Kidney Well II now. You can get this product at www.goutwell.com. I try to use it at least every 3 months. A bottle of Kidney Well runs about $60. And every time I ordered Kidney Well I also ordered Alisma. Kidney Well II is made up of 7 herbs: Poria, Alisma, Rehmannia, Ganoderma, Astragalus, Cyperus and Dioscorea in very specific ratios and concentrations that have shown very positive effects for chronic kidney diseases. To me it seems like a strong kidney cleanser. It sure has had a positive effect on my kidneys; especially in lowering my creatinine and BUN and metabolism of potassium. But with the price being about $10 daily to take it, I can only afford to take it about every 2-3 months.

That investment will certainly do you some real good and far more for your money than what any doctor can do for you. If you hadn't realized it yet...no doctor has ever done a thing to help my kidneys get better; except for Dr. Henry Allen and Dr. David Moskowitz. It's all been about my blood pressure. That's the only help I got from them besides the lab results.

At my first visit to a doctor in 25 years in October 2006, one of the tests they did was an EKG. It had revealed that I also had some heart problems. The main one was that I had an enlarged heart. That is what was causing me to be short of breath quite often. Even when our band was practicing I had to stop in the middle of some songs because I was having too much trouble breathing. I was told it would most likely only get worse and that it might get a little better if I was lucky. Holy crap! Was I shocked at that information! But once I felt I had my creatinine under control after doing so for 3 years, I asked Dr. Allen to do another EKG. I drove about 15 miles to another office of White River Rural Health and had the EKG done.

I asked for this because of how my blood pressure was always high any time anyone in the medical profession took it. An EKG would show that I had an enlarged heart if my blood pressure had been high for most or a lot of the time. Dr. Allen told me my EKG was "good". I asked if that was good, real good, or just OK. He said it was really good, and that I didn't have any heart problems, including an enlarged heart. I was quite relieved at that. And when I went to the ER for that false potassium test result, they did another EKG. That was about 10 months after the one I just told you about; my second EKG. Dr. Allen said it was even better than the one 10 months earlier! Again, I was super satisfied and excited to know I had been doing a great job of controlling my blood pressure and curing my enlarged heart condition. You might ask "How did you do that?"

What I CAN tell you is this... I made a habit of taking Co-Q10, magnesium and fish oil. Co-Q10 helps make your veins and arteries more elastic. So when high blood pressure exerts higher pressure within your circulatory system, your veins and arteries are much less likely to tear or explode, thus causing a stroke or a heart attack. Also, magnesium not only cures and prevents bladder stones, kidney stones and bone spurs, it causes your heart to relax. Calcium causes your heart to contract, while magnesium causes your heart to relax. This combined activity is known as your pulse or heartbeat. Uh huh! So if you've got heart arrhythmia or any other problems concerning any abnormalities in your heart beat, magnesium may very well cure that problem for you.

The fish oil allows your blood to flow more smoothly and efficiently throughout your body, as well as oiling those arthritic joints and giving you a heaping helping dose of omega-3. I recommend 250mg magnesium and 1000mg fish oil most days for everyone. I have yet to have anyone tell me where they're getting their proper daily dose of magnesium, and are also hard pressed to tell me where they are getting any omega-3! So it's almost certain that you are deficient in both omega-3 and magnesium.

Some Important Facts about all this – I touched on what I was doing from about December 2006 through present day, all the time I have been going to the doctor just like all of you do and are doing. But what I was doing the whole time, day after day after day, week upon weeks, month upon months... the whole four years and more... was doing all the things I told you in Chapters 5,

6 & 7; working to limit, eliminate and avoid the saturation of poisons in our food, drinks and water supply. Ah Ha! Those chapters were about what I was doing habitually and obsessively in those first few years up until now.

Then I took Chapter 8 to tell you about my difficult experiences with those in the medical profession, as I was learning to do the very things I told you about in those first five chapters. I didn't want to inject a bunch of details about how I was always busy working on limiting my intake of poisons every or most steps of my story.

So I got those details out of the way in those first few chapters. It doesn't matter what doctor's visit I talked about, or time of the day, week, month or year, I was always working to keep the poisons OUT of my body, keep eating healthy and drinking that awesome, life giving PURE WATER from our fluoride water filter. The fluoride water filter was the first thing we bought to begin our campaign to reduce the large amounts of poisons we were ingesting.

The shower filter was the second thing we did. Oh what tremendous assets both of those babies are for your health. After all, your body IS...80% water! Oh...do I have to tell you that your body is NOT 80% water plus fluoride plus chlorine!?! Your body is 80% water. So take my advice...get those water filters first! Every time I feel bad or some discomfort...an upset stomach, tired, puny or the likes...I go get my water jug or bottle and start drinking down that awesome PURE WATER! It never fails to help. I cannot even imagine NOT having a fluoride water filter. I can't believe I never thought it was important to have one, much less have a shower filter too!

How many of you realized that during this entire chapter of telling you my experiences with the medical profession, that I never got any help for my kidneys from doctors and the medical profession? The one and only exception to that was Dr. David Moskowitz's treatment.

From day one, the doctors did nothing to help my kidneys. See, your kidneys are responsible for many things for your body. Removing poisons is just one of those tasks. So with all the saturation of poisons in everything, your kidneys get overloaded and become soaked with the excess poisons. Your kidneys turn to mush and begin to fail. Of course, I didn't know this before I had chronic kidney disease. With 30 million adults in the US with chronic kidney disease, you'd think someone would care about a cure. I sure do.

So I did what I believed COULD help my kidneys the past four and a half years, without having anyone to tell me IF what I was doing was going to help my kidneys. No one COULD. No one had ever gotten better at the hands of this country's common medical profession. But regardless of how willfully incompetent doctors are about curing diseases, I still had to find a way to cure myself or at least get better. And while I was doing everything to help my kidneys, I got some near miraculous surprises:

I cured myself of arthritis – What do I mean exactly? I had arthritis for at least 20 years. Most of that time I would have swollen painful joints 4 or 5 days every week. But after going cold turkey on the sodas and fruit juices for a few months, I noticed I wasn't hardly getting any swollen, painful joints. I had been taking Glucosamine a lot. But when I started taking fish oil regularly at that time, those swollen, painful red joints disappeared.

And to this day, I still haven't had any arthritis. I'm going on six years without arthritis. Doctors say arthritis is NOT curable. I cured myself merely by taking magnesium oxide and vitamin C. Can you GUESS if I believe that! LOL I am so thankful that I don't!

I cured myself of heartburn, acid reflux – What do I mean exactly? I had acid reflux for at least 20 years too. I had heartburn pretty much all the time. I had heartburn at least 4 or 5 times a day that I HAD to take some TUMS for immediately! I got to where I would take those little anti-acid tablets to get some relief. You take those to prevent heartburn. But even though I took them every day, I still had heartburn, but not as much. I still had heartburn daily. But while I was concentrating on finding something that would help my kidneys, my heartburn came to an end. I took apple cider vinegar for some bouts of heartburn for a few months after starting the crusade to avoid the poisons in our food, drinks and water. But after that my heartburn went away.

I cured myself of headaches – What do I mean exactly? For the past 20 years or so I have had headaches. I didn't have any when I was a kid or teenager that I can remember. But into my early twenties, I started getting headaches every once and awhile. As the years have gone by I just accepted that headaches were normal. Everyone gets them. Some people MORE. Some people LESS. But just a few months into the start of my poison crusade, just like the arthritis and heartburn, the headaches faded away. I was so busy trying to save my own life, with death coming soon, that I was only concerned about helping my kidneys get better; so I didn't have to die or start dialysis in 2008. I never did anything with the intent of curing anything besides chronic kidney disease! But I was greatly surprised at being cured of all this. But hey… there's more!

I cured myself of dandruff – I thought only Head and Shoulders cured dandruff! No, I don't think they make that claim. But dandruff is a common thing too. I use to have dandruff flakes on the shoulders of my shirts all the time. I could shake or brush my hair and watch the flakes fly in the air. I noticed that about other people too, but never said anything to anyone; since dandruff was so common. But barely two months passed after we got our shower filter and my dandruff was all but gone completely!

I look back and say "Of course you have dandruff. You're soaking your scalp with that chlorinated water that destroys the oils in your skin, scalp and hair!" It's pretty much unavoidable unless you use a shower filter. And doing that also cured me of the red, itchy spots on my body I always got and irritated every time I took a shower. This also cured my wife of the same thing and dandruff. Just think of how much money we've saved with the greatly lower use of all the dandruff shampoos and skin lotions?

We always thought dandruff was normal and never could find anything to stop those red, itchy places on our bodies! No one told me these things. I learned them and proved them by personal experiences.

I cured myself of gout – I didn't have gout for 20 years daily like the other diseases and conditions I just mentioned. I had one gout attack about 10 years ago and didn't have another one until about 3 or 4 years ago. It lasted for about two weeks, then went away without me doing anything specifically about gout. Dr. Henry Allen gave me medication to take if I thought I was getting gout again. I used those pills once right after that two month episode with gout in September and October of 2009, and then took one pill on two future occasions shortly after that, but never developed gout again.

Getting back on the high fructose corn syrup brought me two months of gout every day all day. But once I got back OFF the high fructose corn syrup, the gout went away and stayed away. Boy am I glad. It was this that sealed the deal for eternity about high fructose corn syrup being the toxic addicting poison that it is.

The thing that finally ended my gout was me adding pH drops to my drinking water and drinking baking soda and water. I got the pH drops off Ebay. A two months' supply is only about $8. Baking soda is 89¢ for a 1 lb. Box; making it medicinal gold. All disease has to have an acidic environment to exist. So by drinking highly alkaline water, water with baking soda or pH drops, you begin to neutralize the acid that causes all disease.

One great fact that you must learn is that these corporations put these poisons in their products mainly to addict you to their products and turn you into a robot consumer. What I mean by robot consumer is that you buy these poison saturated products and stuff them down your throat and never consider what you're doing…poisoning yourself and creating sickness inside your body. Is THIS what you really want to do? I don't really think so.

So why do you do it again and again, day after week after month, year in year out? It's because your mind has a craving for those poisons. You ate some food item saturated with poisons and even though it didn't nourish your body as real food does, that food or drink gave your body sensations as those poisons were damaging your body. I hope I remembered to repeat these facts during this book.

This is where you gain the victory over those poisons…in your mind; as you are eating or drinking these poison saturated foods and drinks. Does the food or drinks nourish you, or are you eating and drinking those products because you have a craving for them in your head? I talked about this earlier, about using this information to see if you like whole milk or are addicted to the drugs and chemicals in the milk's fat.

I cured myself of bleeding gums – This was another big surprise to me. My gums had been bleeding a lot for about 15-20 years prior to my kidneys failing. It got to where every time I brushed my teeth, my gums would start bleeding in front and then in other places; turning my sudsy white toothpaste into pink sudsy toothpaste every time. I lost some teeth from this too. And all this time I was brushing my teeth 6 or 7 times every day. I brushed after I ate or drank anything. But my gums bled every time in spite of this excess brushing habit of mine.

But, just like the heartburn, headaches, arthritis and other chronic conditions I had for up to twenty years had faded away during the first six months of my poison elimination crusade, my gums stopped bleeding. They stopped bleeding for a few months before I was willing to believe my gums might not bleed again. And over the four years since they first stopped bleeding, my gums haven't bled at all from brushing. The only time my gums bleed now is when I puncture them or cut them with a dental pick. You know, one of those hook shaped metal tooth picks on a 6 inch plastic stick/handle. My gums have firmed up, and my teeth have too. My gums gave me the visual for what my kidneys must have looked like when they failed…mushy and soft and slowly disintegrating.

I have also all but cured myself of chronic kidney disease. My last blood tests revealed that I am closer than ever. **I also prevented myself from developing diabetes.** The doctors were always looking for that and said that almost all patients with chronic kidney disease develop diabetes. No doubt, I teetered on the edge of diabetes sometimes, but did specific things to try and prevent that. You'll be surprised at what I learned to help my pancreas to prevent diabetes. I also cured myself of other conditions like internal intestinal bleeding; and bladder stones which I had for several years back in the mid 90's. But what I have achieved with my kidneys seems to make me a pioneer in curing chronic kidney disease. I know I could have done a better job and still can. But I was too busy DOING all these things to see IF and WHAT helped, if anything. So I had to have it proven to me for an extended period of time before I could talk about any of this being a cure.

Hey, it might have just been a normal break from headaches, heartburn and/or arthritis. No one told me any of this would cure anyone. And I searched the INTERNET and quizzed every nurse and doctor I've ever come into contact with about any cures for these things! Or maybe there's a powerful conspiracy against just ME, to make sure I am the ONLY one who never gets to hear these alleged "cures" the rest of you already know? Let me know IF you have any proof of that! LOL I would like to save your life and have you avoid most sickness and suffering. But only YOU can do that for yourself and your family. **This book gives you the information to guide you in doing just that.**

I went ahead and wrote this book so that people could prevent all these diseases and cure them too. I am not saying I have the complete story on cures and preventions. But I do know I am telling you the most important things to do, and the most powerful things to do, and the most important things NOT to do...to change your health in the most positive ways you never thought possible.

I am not some author who came up with a new subject for my next book I wish to market! I am the guy who became the only person in my area of my state and maybe the whole state and country, that got better after being diagnosed with chronic kidney disease; and did so by doing things I had to learn and prove in order to save my own life. These are my credentials. This is my proof of how I proved I could do what this country's modern medical profession could not and/or would not do...help a person with chronic kidney disease(CKD) get better! So even if you only have CKD caused by hypertension, doing what I set forth in this book will delay dialysis for years and very possibly avoid dialysis altogether.

Even if I started getting worse now, I wouldn't need dialysis until early 2014; SIX YEARS after doctors said I would be on dialysis. So far I've saved nearly $300,000 in medical bills. That's about $50,000 without counting the $100,000 a year for dialysis. Now if this idea catches on, the health-care crisis will end real fast! The millions of bankruptcies over medical bills would end and your suffering would greatly diminish. The food companies won't change until you refuse to buy their poisons, by reading the labels while you're in the grocery store and never putting that garbage in your basket to bring it home.

For now, you all have to do this for yourselves, since We the People have no government to do this for us. FDA approved safe...still killing us by the tens of thousands yearly, because the concept of poisons being bad hinders corporate profits. **You won't knock the chip off my shoulder! It got glued on when they tried to poison me to death.**

My Personal Perspective

I had set out to do something and some things to try and help my kidneys get better so I could avoid dialysis, or at least delay dialysis and maybe save my life. I never had any intention of writing a book about any of this. I also never set out to cure myself of anything but chronic kidney disease. After all, doctors said I would be dead no later than 2009 unless I got a successful kidney transplant. And that was only a possibility! No doctors had done anything to help my kidneys. So it was all up to me to help myself if I was going to get any help for my kidneys.

Now what is so troubling about doctors is that I went to them for help and a cure. But even though I went to the doctor again and again and again…I never got one bit of help for my kidneys! **How the heck does anyone expect doctors to help them when doctors won't even as much as TRY to do anything to help your kidneys when you are diagnosed with chronic kidney disease!**

All they do is preach death and dialysis while they hold your hand and lead you to your grave without any hope or cure; in order to maximize their income. And do so without any regard for your life or your health. This willful incompetence is THE WAY of the medical profession when it comes to sickness and disease. I wish it was not true. But it is.

What I did to help my kidneys has proven to be unknown among doctors and the medical profession. You can NOT learn how to get better with chronic kidney disease from doctors. You can't get a cure for arthritis, headaches, acid reflux, gout, diabetes or even the common cold from the medical profession. All my help for my kidneys came from myself. And I proved that what I had done actually worked, and did so with proof that no doctor has denied.

I'm alive right now because of what I learned in just the past 5 years. This is my story about how I saved my own life and cured myself. And if you want to do the same, this book is your only hope. And you are hearing from the horse's mouth, how the horse saved his own life, doing the things that the horse had to learn and prove while waiting to die, in order for the horse to save his own life. And I did it!

So maybe you are one of those who loses his car keys and looks on the TV and doesn't find them, and then does what no one is doing about their own health and lives…you look elsewhere until you find those keys.

So, as the doctors give you NO CURES when you go to them…LOOK ELSEWHERE for a cure and you'll find it!

9 - More Help for Your Kidneys and Diabetes, Gout & Heart Disease

Everything I did the past five years was centered on my chronic kidney disease. I have tried all kinds of things. Most of them helped. A few did not help. The best thing for kidney disease is pure water. So start with a fluoride water filter as I pointed out in the Poisons in Your Water chapter. Drink 1 ounce of water for every 2 pounds of body weight. Drinking water is the best way to wash and cleanse your insides. But drinking water with chlorine and fluoride is almost enough to negate the positive effects water has on your kidneys and whole body. So at least get a carbon water filter to filter out 90% of the chlorine and no fluoride! They only cost $20-30.

Making sure you hold your blood pressure down is essential, and your doctor will tell you this. Take Hawthorn berries, L-Arginine, Fish oil, magnesium, B6 and garlic to help lower your blood pressure naturally, in addition to your prescribed medicines. Even apple cider vinegar can lower your blood pressure. It's high in vitamins that are helpful for lowering blood pressure, like Vitamins C, A, E, B1, B2 and B6, as well as potassium, magnesium and copper. Apple Cider Vinegar is alkaline, so it improves your body's pH levels. Valerian Root helps to calm you and lower blood pressure, but should be taken with caution and only according to directions. Dealing with stress goes a long way in controlling your blood pressure. So make sure you take measures to minimize your stress.

It is my opinion that you are best off taking Clonidine and Quinapril to control blood pressure artificially. Taking Atenolol only slows down your heartbeat to minimize the number of times your heart beats. But doesn't actually lower your blood pressure. You could also take a CCB, Calcium Channel Blocker, but only do so for about a year at a time, since doing so any longer causes your PTH glands to release Calcium from your bones and weaken them. Due to the damage to your kidneys, which makes hormones to control your blood pressure, drugs to control blood pressure are almost always needed. This is the one area I am still working on to correct. But I think it may take some artificial means of reversing the DNA or gene damage that caused this high blood pressure in the first place.

The best thing I found to help my kidneys was a concentrated Chinese herbal product called Kidney Well. I always use Kidney Well and Alisma together. But you can get products from the same company for whatever your chronic kidney disease is. For their great kidney products visit their web site at: http://www.goutwell.com/kidney.html I use Kidney Well as often as I can; which is at least every 2-3 months. It always helps. I usually take anywhere from 6-10 tablets of Kidney Well and 2-3 capsules of Alisma per dose 3 times daily on an empty stomach. It's good to take one of those doses right before bed time. There are no side effects to this herbal remedy, except for some light stomach pains or discomfort occasionally. It gives you a clean feeling.

When it comes to holding down your protein, I have found that red meat is the hardest on your kidneys. So it was easy for me to get off red meat and just eat omega-3 rich fish, and chicken and turkey. You should take Bromelain with meals that include meat. Bromelain breaks down protein real well, and is a natural product made from pineapple. Bromelain is also good at flushing excess protein out of your kidneys; a common problem for those with chronic kidney disease. Using Bromelain and papaya enzyme helps take the load off your pancreas in its role in digestion; which helps prevent diabetes. Be sure to follow the instructions to cure Diabetes, since **Diabetes is the cause of 90% of kidney patients reaching end stage renal failure.**

I drank gallons of Goji, Noni and Mangosteen Juice and ate Goji berries over the time since first being diagnosed with chronic kidney disease. Regardless of any rumors of these being miracle cures, the extremely high anti-oxidant properties was reason enough to use these juices and berries. The problem is finding the rare few pure juices.

Stop cooking with the microwave. Only use the microwave oven to heat things, but only for 30 seconds or less. The damage cooking in a microwave does to food turns a good meal into a bad meal for your health. Microwaving food destroys up to 97% of the delicate vitamins and phytonutrients, plant medicines, in food.

If your doctor tries to trick you with white lies about your PTH hormone levels being high, and you are on a CCB, Calcium channel blocker, like Amlodipine, then simply ask your doctor to take you off the calcium channel blocker and switch it to an ACE inhibitor such as Quinapril, aka Accupril. Your Parathyroid glands control calcium levels in your body. Once your Parathyroid glands sense that the calcium channel blocker is blocking calcium to your heart, your Parathyroid glands will begin to release hormones, PTH. This causes your system to start releasing calcium from your bones into your blood stream to make up for that "simulated" calcium deficiency. Doctors only want you to do another drug to control the side effects of the first drug, the calcium channel blocker.

Avoid taking Ibuprofen, naproxen and aspirin. All of these are hard on your kidneys. If you work on avoiding poisons, the need for any of these over the counter drugs will become a thing of the past. Tylenol is hard on your liver. I have only taken a few Aleve in the past 5 years, and that was for severe tooth or back pain.

Your big problem is usually controlling your potassium. Potassium is in just about everything you eat, but is highest in beans and peas; especially green beans. So I rarely eat any beans or peas. 8 ounces of beans has as much potassium as 3 or 4 oranges or bananas. I never eat more than 2 oranges or bananas in a day. One of each is as far as I go. Cutting down on meat portions will help limit protein and potassium too. Eating cheese and drinking milk and orange juice should be held to a minimum if you want to control your potassium. Eight ounces of milk or orange juice contains around 300mg of potassium which is the same amount of potassium in one medium orange or banana. One thing I have noticed is that even when I eat potassium rich fruits, it doesn't seem to have the potassium raising effect that meats have.

So lean toward eating fresh fruits and vegetables. I wish we could get watermelon year round. I am always thrilled to eat good watermelon. It is nothing but good for you. It is a great source of distilled water. A funny thing that is true is that if you really want the best detox program for your body, eat watermelon and soak in a hot tub as much as you can. Cantaloupe is great for the same reasons. You will notice how you have to pee more often after eating either one too.

There aren't really any vitamins I take just for the kidneys. But I do take vitamins and herbs that do help my kidneys such as fish and flax seed oil, Taurine, Vitamin C, Vitamin E, B-Complex, L-Arginine, Astragalus and bilberry. And the Kidney Well is a formula of about 5 herbs; which includes Astragalus and Alisma. But make sure you steer clear of herbs like Licorice Root and Celery Seed. You can take Celery Seed as a diuretic as long as you are sure that your kidneys are not inflamed. Taking amino acids, B-Complex, will provide those B Vitamins you'll lose by restricting your protein consumption.

You can read Dr. Mackenzie Walser's book titled Coping With Kidney Disease: A 12-Step Program to Avoid Dialysis. His book gives you detailed information and instructions on restricting your protein intake. He kept lots of people off dialysis for years by putting his patients on protein restricted diets. He was a doctor and professor at the well-known John Hopkins Medical Center and University. His book was the only help I got from a doctor before I met Dr. Moskowitz.

You should also read Chapter 3 and see what Dr. Moskowitz says about getting on his treatment program. As long as your creatinine isn't above 3.9, Dr. Moskowitz can probably keep you off dialysis. And even if your creatinine is above 3.9, he is still willing to try and help you. Between his treatment and what I did to help my kidneys, as told in this book, I do not know of a single other thing that can help anyone with chronic kidney disease. But hey…the entire medical profession can't and does not do a thing to help the kidneys of chronic kidney disease patients. They only treat the symptoms of CKD while they hold your hand and lead you to the dialysis machine and the grave.

Another disease that is common among people with kidney disease is:

Gout - Gout is an extremely painful condition. Gout is caused by an overproduction and over population of uric acid. Uric acid has needle-like points on the crystals. The pain of gout is caused by those needle-like crystals. Just imagine tens of thousands of needles inside your big toe or ankle, and you get the idea behind what gout is doing to you. Although most gout attacks are the result of consumption of high fructose corn syrup, especially in liquid form such as fruit juices and soda pops, gout is also caused by other things. The common factor among all the causes is the introduction of poisons or some other body trauma such as chemotherapy, joint injury and dehydration.

This tells you that drinking lots of pure water will help gout. And working on avoiding poisons in your food and drinks will cure your gout, and/or prevent gout altogether. Drinking too much alcohol can bring on a gout attack. Alcohol is mostly a sugar, and a poison to your body. Drinking beer and eating shrimp together are known to cause gout.

I cured myself of gout by getting off the high fructose corn syrup. And I nailed this fact down forever. I went through a phase for 2 to 3 months where I was tired of being laughed at and hated on because of my speaking out against high fructose corn syrup. So, I just gave it up and decided that since I'm so crazy for speaking out against high fructose corn syrup...I would now shut my fucking mouth and never do it again. And since, according to most everyone else, high fructose corn syrup is only a poison in MY crazy opinion, then it was perfectly safe for me to consume high fructose corn syrup.

I stopped trying to avoid high fructose corn syrup for 2-3 months. Then I got gout, and had gout all day every day for two whole months! And that is what broke me and stood me up against high fructose corn syrup FOREVER! I mean this one is nailed down! But, to test this "opinion" of mine one final time, I told myself I would stay off the high fructose corn syrup, UNLESS I had another gout attack AFTER getting off the high fructose corn syrup again. It's been 2 years since that last gout attack, so I know it's the high fructose corn syrup.

But you really need to work on avoiding poisons as this book explains, and do things to boost your immune system like taking Astragalus. Avoiding aluminum based anti-deodorants will help too, by keeping your lymph system healthy. Once that aluminum soaks into your underarm, it poisons your lymph glands and nodes. Your lymph system is part of your immune system.

If you just have to use drugs, ask your doctor to prescribe you Colchicine. It is taken when you feel a gout attack coming on. Otherwise, you'll be taking gout medication every day to prevent gout until you can get yourself completely cured.

Another thing you can do to cure yourself of Gout, even if you've done everything you know to do so far, is to drink high alkaline water. To create high alkaline water, it's best to use filtered water from a fluoride filter or osmosis water filtration system, then add some pH drops to that filtered water. The filters take out all that acidic chlorine and fluoride and other toxins. That removes the bitter taste of tap water and your water's pH becomes 7.0 or so; which is alkaline. Then if you add pH drops to that filtered water, the pH rises to 7.5 – 8.0 or so. Drinking 1 ounce of high alkaline water per 2 pounds of body weight daily will soon reverse the acidic state that you slowly put your body in over the years. It is more economical to just drink ½ teaspoon baking soda with 4-6 ounces of water 2-5x a day to cure your gout and all diseases.

This ripe for disease acidic state is created by regular consumption of animal products and sugars. Face the facts. Gout is the effect of overproduction of Uric ACID crystals. Did you get that? Uric ACID! And of course, those crystals rely on that acidic state to survive and multiply. That high alkaline water goes right through your kidneys! And as it does, it reverses the acidic state of your kidneys. And as your kidneys slowly create the contents of your blood, those contents that become your blood, flow throughout your entire body; alkalizing your entire body over time.

Depending on how many animal products and sugar you continue to consume, you should reverse the acidic state of your body in 3 or 4 months on average. And the gout just fades away and becomes just a memory! Another problem kidney patients usually face is heart disease.

Heart disease – Basically, you need to take magnesium and fish oil. Flax seed oil is also good for the heart. Your heart needs calcium to contract and magnesium to relax your heart. This produces normal heart rhythms. Take 250-400mg daily for a few weeks if you haven't already been taking magnesium tablets. Then go to a maintenance dose of 250-400mg every other day or every few days.

Co-Q10 helps make your veins and arteries more elastic, which helps cure hardening of the arteries. Fish oil produces the same effect by emulsifying the fats and plaque that build up in your arteries and promote atherosclerosis. Take 100-150mg Co-Q10 daily, and at least 1000mg fish or flax seed oil daily. Fish oil and flax seed oil help your heart and blood pressure because they contain omega-3 fatty acid. Fish oil helps improve circulation. Omega-3 also reduces sudden death from cardiac arrhythmias. Fish oil also reduces triglycerides levels and helps stabilize blood clotting mechanisms; which prevents blood clots, a major cause of heart attacks and strokes. Fish oil "thins" the blood.

Niacin helps clean out your veins and arteries of plaque and other debris in your blood. Taking fish oil and niacin can cure heart disease caused by plaque and hardening of the arteries. You need to take large doses of niacin to do this, but you run into a peculiar problem known as the red flush. Red flush is caused by doses of niacin as low as 25mg. This red flush is caused by the niacin expanding your capillaries to twice their normal size; allowing more blood flow to the surface of the skin. Be glad when you get it! This is the proof of the niacin working. By expanding your capillaries, your blood is able to carry a lot of toxins out of your body. To increase your dose of niacin, do this:

Start with 25mg niacin 2-3 times a day. When you no longer get the red flush, increase the dose to 50mg 2-3 times a day. Repeat this until you are at 100mg 2-3 times a day. Then up the dose by 50mg each time until you no longer get the red flush. You can do this all the way up to 500mg. Just remember that if you stop taking niacin for a while, don't start back taking the same dose as you were. The red flush could very well be painful instead of warming and slightly uncomfortable.

When I was first diagnosed with chronic kidney disease, my EKG showed that I had an enlarged heart. I had trouble breathing more than a few times in those months just prior to and after that EKG. Doctors only expected it to get worse, not better. Because of the way I have eaten the past 30 years, I don't have a problem with cholesterol. But I cured myself of an enlarged heart by doing the same things I told you here and getting rid of the poisons I was consuming. I asked Dr. Allen if I could get another EKG to see if I had damaged my heart by having long term high blood pressure. My EKG was very good. Just a few months ago I had an EKG again and it was almost perfect.

Be sure to do things for Stress to help minimize putting harmful pressure on your heart and circulatory system. And of course, exercise regularly, drink lots of pure water and eat as many fresh fruits and vegetables as you can. And, since people often mistake heartburn (acid reflux) as a heart attack, be sure to use Apple Cider Vinegar to cure your heartburn, Acid Reflux.

Cardiovascular disease is the leading cause of death in the USA, even though most heart disease is preventable. Use this book to help you do so.

And do I have to tell you to stop smoking or stop drinking alcohol? These are the only 2 poisons that doctors will warn you about. If you gotta drink, don't drink in excess. That means, no more than 2 ounces in a 24 hour period, no more than 3 or 4 times a week. Alcohol is acidic and cigarettes are packed with poisons. I just went ahead and mentioned this in case some of you might tell yourself it's OK to smoke cigarettes and drink alcohol if I didn't mention it.

So that's about it for the information you need to avoid dialysis and most likely cure yourself of kidney disease and the diseases that develop as a result of the progression of your chronic kidney disease. And for the things I need to say to you before The End of this book comes, I have included the next Chapter titled **My Final Words.**

My Final Words

Well, here we are at the very end of the book. I accomplished what I set out to do when I first started writing this book. I actually did a whole lot better job than I thought I would. I didn't want to sound preachy or that I was on a pedestal talking down to you. I really just wanted to share with as many people as I could, about the incredible journey I went on once my kidneys blew out in late 2006.

I never set out to cure myself of arthritis, gout, headaches or anything. I only wanted to try and help my kidneys get better to avoid going on dialysis and dying. I cured myself of every disease I had. So what I did cured every disease and medical condition I had, except for high blood pressure.

The damage to my kidneys caused my kidneys to stop releasing hormones that help control blood pressure. Everything is fixed, and I have eliminated at least 90% of the poisons that I didn't even call poisons until the end of 2006 going into 2007. So I put all the information I needed to cure myself of all those diseases and medical conditions in this book. And **90% of this book came from my memory in my head, because I know all this stuff so well.**

This is where I would use some catchy little sales pitch and tell you that IF this book does not improve your health, you can have a complete refund! But there are a lot of things in this book that will improve your health and save you lots and lots of suffering, inactivity and a whole lot of money. If you really think the problem is the book, then you missed the whole point of the book.

The problem is YOU. It's you that stuffed all those poisons down your throat. There is no condemnation here. It's called accepting responsibility for what you do. You ARE responsible for stuffing that sick crap down your throat. And you can stop it. 100% guaranteed.

Who's gonna stop you? Has anyone stuffed food down your throat by force? Or are you the only one stuffing anything down your throat! And when you take responsibility for what you do, then you'll get that chip on your shoulder at the grocery store against any and every product that is packed with poisons, and leave them on the shelf and out of your basket, so they'll stay out of your home and out of your body.

I don't mean to burden you with all this extra responsibility you have to take on to save your lives and avoid chronic diseases and medical conditions. I wish we had a government in this country. If we did, they would see to it that We, the People are protected from poisons. But they only seek the approval of corporations' ability to make money.

Your health is irrelevant to them. Neither the government nor the corporations will take responsibility for the obligations of their positions. And the excuse is always greed. They're like the sickos in the music industry. If you can sell 100,000 units, but add near naked women to the cover, you can boost your sales to at least 150-175,000. So, they add the naked women and ship it out to market.

And...add high fructose corn syrup to the product and your sales go up 25%. So hey, that CAN'T be bad, because they're making money off it! So the responsibility falls on YOU to learn how to avoid those poisons and eliminate them or at least greatly limit them. Otherwise, you honestly don't have a chance in this country. You can only get one chronic disease after another, and try to find a way to cope with all the pain and suffering.

We live under the bullshit idea that we all gotta get sick to die. So we stand on that bullshit as an excuse why there's no hope of being cured and no way of avoiding disease. And it's all bullshit.

So many of you dread the idea of the doctor telling you that you that you have some deadly chronic disease like kidney disease or cancer. It just doesn't have to be like that. But you can't be making excuses about putting so many poisons in your body. Even though they are FDA certified "safe" doesn't mean poisons are now safe. It means the FDA is full of shit! They should be called the Federal Death Association, not Food and Drug Administration!

You just gotta snap out of it and stop trusting the food, drinks and water to BE, safe! Almost none of it is. And don't expect any of this to change. It won't. You can't expect different results from the same actions. Your poison saturated food, drinks and water are FDA approved and safe.

This book is your chance to change all of that for yourself and touch the lives of so many people with help they never expected, or only expected if a doctor could do it. When I look back at what I did to myself with all the "safe" poison soaked sodas and fruit juice...I am shocked at my own behavior. Not a one of you would've called it odd or wrong. Most actually believed I was eating very healthy. And I was!

But what I was DRINKING blew my kidneys out! I had spent a lot of time over the years making the effort to eat right. I started eating whole wheat bread in 1981. But it wasn't enough to keep me from getting a major chronic disease. I had already accepted the headaches and heartburn as common. And I also never expected any of it to go away permanently.

I started my phase into chronic kidney disease with no hope for a future and the end of my life in sight just 2-3 years away, and with my headaches, arthritis, gout, bleeding gums, dandruff, red itchy spots on my skin, intestinal bleeding and chronic heartburn. And I came out of it completely cured of all of it, and my kidneys healed almost back to normal. If I had a book like this I might've avoided the kidney disease altogether. Hey! If only someone would've told me WATCH WHAT YOU DRINK, I might have avoided it altogether too.

But if this had not of happened, you wouldn't be reading this book right now, and you would have no hope of being cured; much less actually be cured after all the doctors told you there was no hope. I can't tell you that story. I didn't live it that way. Mine is the one where if my life was going to be saved, I HAD to do it. It wasn't going to happen depending on doctors. What I did worked, and I am the one that is the most pleased that it did.

I would love to hear any testimonials from those who cured themselves or had their conditions improve because of what you learned from this book and put to use.

I want to thank my dear wife Sandra for all her support. This book is dedicated to her. The things I have learned that cured me have also prevented her from getting any kind of disease. I am confident of the validity of what I have stated in this book. I am confident in the ability of the information to add years to the lives of those who read this book and put it to use.

The Facebook page for this book is:
www.facebook.com/AvoidingDialysis

Go there to keep up with the book and its impact on people.

DISCLAIMER

This book was written to guide people in doing the things that will improve their health and cure them if they are willing to do the natural things it takes to do so. While there are some facts stated in here that are critical of some things, there is absolutely no intent to defame or misrepresent the facts about these persons, companies or others.

On the contrary, I intentionally left out the names of the companies saturating our food, drinks and water supplies. I did this so that no one would think that talking to these people or companies is of any real value. So, if anyone takes anything said in this book to mean to defame, misrepresent or anything of that nature, they are only stating their opinion of what is in the book, but not stating an opinion based on facts.

I am fully aware of how the people in the medical profession, generally and according to my own experiences, will attack and criticize anything that is not something they do and make money off of. I have no interest in their drama and choose to avoid it altogether. I have never told anyone to stop going to the doctor.

On the contrary, I tell them to cure themselves WHILE they still do what the doctors say for them to do. I'm not afraid of doctors. I just know not to look to doctors or the medical profession for cures.

No one should, in any way, take anything stated in this book as promoting or even suggesting any type of action toward any part of government, companies or the likes.

On the contrary, I suggest you stop buying products with the disease causing poisons pointed out in this book. And no one should be so twisted and perverted in their minds to claim that Individuals do not have the Right to protect ourselves from disease causing poisons and all poisons.

This book places absolutely ZERO HOPE that food companies will ever make the choices to remove the poisons from their products. So, the only choice we have is to freely share the knowledge individuals need to avoid the poisons in food and drink products.

Just because doctors and the rest of the medical profession don't get to make money off the diseases I cure or prevent and never have, doesn't constitute any illegal or inappropriate act or acts.

There are only a rare few places in this book where any text was copied from a web site and pasted into this book. These few places were from Public sites with no copyright stated. This was only done for accuracy of rules and policies.

Anyone who thinks their copyright has been violated in any way, can contact me for a quick and amicable solution in your favor.

Alphabetical Index

Lightning Source UK Ltd.
Milton Keynes UK
UKHW05f1234040518
322083UK00013B/260/P